11 <u>95</u>

S0-ATT-471

Critics Praise *DIET FOR TRANSCENDENCE*
(Previously published as *FOOD FOR THE SPIRIT*)

"*Food For The Spirit* ...makes it clear that all religions teach compassion and that not eating meat is much more than just a healthy way to eat. It is the basis of a profound spiritual life."

—*Hinduism Today*

"The Western world has produced few books on vegetarianism and religion. Therefore, Steven Rosen's book, written from a vegetarian perspective, is a welcome effort....Those who already are vegetarians will be further bolstered in their beliefs."

—*Vegetarian Times*

"To those in whom a concept of universal compassion and awareness of the sacred nature of all creation is still somewhat of a radical concept, Rosen's book will certainly be educational. For others who are already committed to following a path of spiritual growth, and have discovered that being a vegetarian is a major step along this road, this book offers reinforcement and inspiration."

—*On the Issues, Vol. III*

"This wonderful book provides a real service, covering the whole range of reasons for changing to vegetarianism...and one can incorporate as part of that intentionality the theosophical perspective that all life—human and non-human alike—is related in an interdependent whole."

—*The American Theosophist*

"In this book Steven Rosen has recalled the followers of all the world religions to their vegetarian roots. We now have scientific evidence that vegetarianism is good for the body. The greatest spiritual teachers have always known that it is good for the soul."

—Rev. Alvin V. P. Hart,
Episcopal Priest and Hospital Chaplain,
St. Lukes-Roosevelt Hospital, New York

"Vegetarianism is a way of life that we should all move toward for economic survival, physical well-being and spiritual integrity....As a Catholic priest, I highly recommend this book."

—Father Thomas Berry,
Founder, Riverdale Center of Religious Research,
Former Director, History of Religions Program,
Fordham University, New York

"Judaism is founded on a compassionate way of life and provides a complete philosophy for non-killing in relationship to one's food....We hope this book will be widely read and help to encourage the trend toward a more spiritual outlook in relation to food and, consequently, mankind's outlook in general."

—Philip L. Pick,
President and Founder,
The International Jewish Vegetarian Society,
London Headquarters

"...a book such as *Food For The Spirit* is greatly needed, and the teaching of compassion in Mr. Rosen's book should be embraced by Jew and non-Jew alike."

—Rabbi Joseph H. Gelberman,
Tree of Life Synagogue,
President, The New Seminary,
Founder, The Kabbalah Center, New York

"Existing dietary evidence shows that meat, with its ingrained fats, is harmful as food, and religions such as Islam…have left the choice of food open to an individual's option according to circumstances and environment.…The author of *Food For The Spirit*, Mr. Steven Rosen, knows his subject well enough to help those who would like to change their traditional culinary habits and tastes in favour of vegetarianism."

—Al-Hafiz B.A. Masri,
Retired (Sunni) Imam,
The Shah Jehan Mosque,
Woking, England

"All true believers should read *Food For The Spirit* with an open mind. While it is true that Islam does not traditionally require votaries to abjure the use of flesh-foods, author Rosen, in his scholarly study, shows us another side of our great religion.…Drawing upon the esoteric Sufi tradition, the Holy Qu'ran and the life of the Prophet Mohammed (PBUH), the author makes a convincing case for vegetarianism in Islam. As a result, in fact, I am now de-emphasizing meat products from my own diet!"

—Rashid L.R. Mahmud,
Director, Center for Higher Islamic Studies,
Los Angeles, California

"No practicing Christian, Jew, Buddhist, Hindu or Muslim can ignore the imperative of this inspiring book—that the founders and patriarchs of all these higher religions renounced the killing and eating of our four-footed and feathered kin."

—Roshi Philip Kapleau,
Abbot, The Zen Center,
Rochester, New York
Author, *The Three Pillars of Zen*

"The book entitled *Food For The Spirit* is a most timely addition to the promotion of vegetarianism. Cultivating the thoughts of non-hatred and non-injury and abstaining from killing of any living being are so crucial for an individual's peace, harmony, serenity, concentration and attaining liberation from suffering that the Buddha has included these principles in the Noble Eightfold Path, which is the Fourth Noble Truth in Buddhism."

—Ven. H. Gunaratana Thera,
Director, Washington Buddhist Vihara

"Mr. Rosen has done a splendid job in presenting the merits of vegetarianism in the world religions. Sanskrit (Hindu) literature has endorsed the non-meat diet for millennia. And now Mr. Rosen's work may indeed supply the 'Diet For Transcendence' so much lacking in contemporary society."

—Anant S. Tiwari,
Professor of Sanskrit,
University of Gorakhpur, India

"The Indian community at last has a book that successfully describes its vegetarian heritage. Author Steven Rosen deserves the appreciation of all true Hindus—and that of true believers from all the world's great religions."

—Dr. Vibhakar Mody
Director, Hindu Alliance of America,
Washington, D.C.

"I hope that all those who eat animals and yet consider themselves to be living religious lives will read this book, and that it will lead them to see that the exploitation of animals is incompatible with any religion which professes compassion."

—Peter Singer,
Professor of Philosophy,
Monash University, Australia
Author, *Animal Liberation*

"Mr. Rosen's insightful book could not arrive at a better time. We are just now beginning to see the first stirrings of serious religious concern about the rights of animals here in America. His book will help insure that the religious community is fully aroused from its dogmatic slumber....If animals could talk, they would thank Steven Rosen."

—Tom Regan,
Associate Professor of Philosophy,
North Carolina State University
Author, *The Case for Animal Rights*

Diet For Transcendence

VEGETARIANISM AND THE WORLD RELIGIONS

Diet For
Transcendence

VEGETARIANISM
AND THE WORLD RELIGIONS

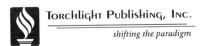 Torchlight Publishing, Inc.

shifting the paradigm

Colorado Christian University
Library
180 S. Garrison
Lakewood, Colorado 80226

Copyright ©1997 by Steven J. Rosen

Previous edition published by Bala Books under the title *Food for the Spirit*, copyright 1987 by Steven J. Rosen

All rights reserved. No part of this book may be reproduced, stored in a retrieval system, or transmitted in any form, by any means, including mechanical, electronic, photocopying, recording, or otherwise, without prior written consent of the publisher.

First Printing 1997

Cover design by Stewart Cannon / Logo Loco Graphics
Printed in the United States of America

Published simultaneously in The United States of America and Canada by Torchlight Publishing

Library of Congress Cataloging-in-Publishing Data
Rosen, Steven
     Diet for transcendence : vegetarianism and the world religions / by Steven Rosen
          p.   cm.
     Originally published: Food for the spirit, New York : Bala Books, 1987
     Includes bibliographical references and index
     ISBN 1-887089-05-5
     1. Vegetarianism — Religious aspects.   I. Title.
BL65.V4R67   1997   97-16123
291.5'693– –dc21

Attention Colleges, Universities, Corporations, Associations and Professional Organizations: *Diet For Transcendence* is available at special discounts for bulk purchases for promotions, premiums, fund-raising or educational use. Special books, booklets, or excerpts can be created to suit your specific needs.

For more information contact the Publisher

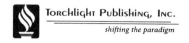

Torchlight Publishing, Inc.
shifting the paradigm

PO Box 52, Badger, CA 93603
Email: torchlight@compuserve.com
1-888-TORCHLT toll free

DEDICATION

To
His Divine Grace
A. C. Bhaktivedanta Swami Prabhupada,
who taught me
to see God
in every living creature.

ACKNOWLEDGMENTS

No one individual could claim exclusive credit for the book you are about to read. Generations of scholars and researchers in the fields of religion and diet have contributed to this work more substantially than I, for to a certain degree I have merely compiled their words and thoughts. The present volume does owe a debt of gratitude, however, to certain individuals who have been particularly helpful.

I would first of all like to thank Mr. Isaac Bashevis Singer, winner of the 1978 Nobel Prize for literature, for having kindly contributed a prefatory essay (which appeared in the original volume). Nathaniel Altman, who was personally responsible for initiating the whole genre of health-and-diet books in the early 1970s with his *Eating for Life*, deserves thanks for his insightful and gracious foreword and his help with the original manuscript. Joshua M. Greene, the original publisher of this book, has inspired me throughout and has done considerable editing on the text as a whole.

I would also like to thank Paul Obis, the publisher and senior editor of *Vegetarian Times*, who commissioned me to write an abbreviated version of the text, which he published in his December 1985 and January 1986 issues. My lifelong friend, Rabbi Richard Schulman, gave me many helpful suggestions, especially in regard to the Judaeo-Christian tradition, and he made sure that my Jewish history was accurate and my Bible translations were clear.

There were many others who helped make this work a reality, including the industrious staff of Bala Books. I would also like to thank Phil Gallelli and family (especially his daughter, Sita), Greg Stein, who encouraged me to update the book, and my new friends at Torchlight, for having the foresight and courage to reprint it. To all the people above (literally and figuratively), I extend my heartfelt appreciation and gratitude.

CONTENTS

FOREWORD

People have been eating animals since at least the Ice Age, when, some anthropologists say, our early ancestors abandoned a plant-oriented diet in favor of one containing meat. The custom of meat-eating has continued to the present day, through necessity (as with the Eskimo), habit, or conditioning. Most of all, the practice has continued due to a lack of awareness.

In the last fifty years, however, recognized authorities in health, nutrition and biochemistry have put forward ample evidence that meat-eating is unnecessary for good health and shown that the carnivorous diet is detrimental to human beings. The documentation for this can be freely researched, and there are many good books extolling the virtues of vegetarianism on scientific grounds.

Moreover, meat-eating today involves—for the animal—a long and cruel process of forced imprisonment, biological manipulation, transportation over long distances in crowded and unsanitary conditions, and finally, violent death in the slaughterhouse. After that, the poor animal's remains are eaten. The average person living today in the United States, Canada or Australia consumes over 200 pounds of meat a year, while per capita meat consumption in Western Europe follows close behind. In order to satisfy our demand for meat, more than four billion cattle, calves, sheep, hogs, chickens, ducks and turkeys are slaughtered each year. During a seventy-year lifetime, the meat consumed by an average American or Canadian involves the slaughter of approximately eleven cattle, one calf, three lambs and sheep, twenty-three hogs, forty-five turkeys, 1,100 chickens and some 862 pounds of fish. The amount of pain inflicted upon these creatures (in order to provide meat for our pleasure) is beyond calculation. In addition, animals raised for slaughter consume huge quantities of valuable grains and legumes—food that could otherwise feed millions of starving people around the world. For these and other reasons, many are turning to vegetarianism. In America alone, there are now some ten million vegetarians.

As the meatless diet has grown in popularity over the years, a number of books have been written on the subject. Some of these explore the health reasons behind vegetarianism and point out how a vegetarian diet can help prevent heart attacks, strokes, cancer and other diseases. Some books focus on the ecological, world food and economic aspects of a meatless diet and show how to enjoy gourmet nutrition without having to spend a lot of money. Others describe how the plant kingdom is the primary source of vital nutrients and how vegetarian diets provide more than enough of the proteins, vitamins and minerals we need each day. Still other books consider many of the ethical, moral and philosophical reasons behind the vegetarian diet. Few works, however, have ever attempted to tackle the difficult subject of vegetarianism and the world religions. *Diet for Transcendence* is the first book to do so with depth and clarity.

Drawing from a wealth of original religious documents and texts, author Steven Rosen takes us on a fascinating journey back in time to explore the essential and often misunderstood roots of the world's major religious traditions, to discover how vegetarianism was a cherished part of their philosophy and practice. He carefully examines and exposes many of the myths about Buddha, Mohammed and Jesus Christ which have long been used to justify meat-eating on religious grounds. *Diet for Transcendence* clearly shows that religious compassion was meant to be all-encompassing, directed toward animals as it is toward humans.

In religious discussion, diet—like sex—is a controversial issue. Unlike other books which are either overly emotional or gloss over important matters of doctrine, *Diet for Transcendence* probes, carefully and logically, the depths of each issue and explores its subject with honesty, clarity and precision. This makes the book easy to read, if also uncomfortable: many of the issues discussed in the following pages are considered sacred and have remained unquestioned by religionists for centuries. Steven Rosen's straightforward examination, based on early manuscripts (as opposed to popular and contemporary translations) and ancient traditions (as distinct from later forms of religious expression), is likely to undermine many dogmatically accepted beliefs and cause a great deal of debate and controversy. *Diet for Transcendence* will give food for thought.

The ideas in this book did not originate with the author. Rather, they are the same truths stressed by spiritual teachers throughout history. Religion has always taught, in essence, that reverence for all life is a high spiritual ideal, and that universal brotherhood is the summit of genuine spirituality. This little volume should go a long way toward establishing these goals.

—Nathaniel Altman, Author, *Eating For Life*

INTRODUCTION

"For that which befalleth the sons of men,
befalleth beasts, even one thing befalleth them:
As the one dieth, so dieth the other.
Yes, they have all one breath. So that a man hath no
pre-eminence above a beast—for all is vanity."

—Ecclesiastes 3:19

Each day thousands of human beings are born, and each day thousands die. At times the world appears to be little more than a vast ocean of birth and death. Animals, too, struggle to remain afloat, and although our activities in life may differ, our end is invariably the same. In terms of mortality, humans and animals are perfect equals.

Human life does of course differ from other forms of life, and this is perhaps best expressed in the human quest for spiritual knowledge. Man's pursuit of God—regardless of the particular tradition—separates him from animals. It is doubtful that an animal will pick up this book, for instance, even for a cursory glance.

Although religions diverge on points of theology and ritual, they unanimously agree on the need for moral codes and ethical principles. Implicit in these codes and principles is the necessity of vegetarianism and compassion for animals. It is the purpose of this book to show that the world's major religious traditions and their earliest adherents were indeed sympathetic toward the meatless way of life and, in many cases, emphasized vegetarianism.

The issue of vegetarianism and religion is itself overshadowed by the religious hypocrisy which preaches brotherhood and human slaughter in the same breath. While mercy and compassion are qualities espoused by all religionists (and many non-religionists), the world's major religions have done

1

little to promote them. Indeed, we inflict violence and prejudice upon our *human* neighbors, even as we direct the same toward the animal world. Religion, in fact, seems to instigate violence rather than eliminate it. The examples are numerous: the Crusades, the Inquisition, the perennial fighting in Northern Ireland between Catholics and Protestants, the endless hostility between the Jews and their Muslim neighbors, the Hindu/Muslim killings in postwar India and the bloodshed of the recent past between Buddhists and Hindus in Sri Lanka. Apparently, despite the spiritual mandate for mercy and compassion, many religions exclude not only animals from their scope, but human beings from other religious traditions as well.

Something is amiss. Ideally, religious temperament should run counter to intolerance. The qualities of love, mercy and compassion—the avowed goals of all the major religious traditions—are extolled, and hate, violence and prejudice are condemned. While this is what religions preach in theory, in practice this has rarely been the case. As noted, some of history's bloodiest battles have been fought on religious grounds. While this, in and of itself, does not invalidate organized religion, it makes us question how effectively religious institutions practice what they preach. If those who implement religion—the leaders, philosophers, theologians and avowed adherents—are confused about the treatment of people from other religious traditions, could they then not also be confused about the treatment of animals? Have they perhaps drawn artificial limits on the scope of mercy?

While such limits are evident today, earlier forms of religion had a different story to tell. In fact, the further back we go in religious history, the more respect we find for life in all its forms. Quite naturally, vegetarianism played a part in this respect for all life. Islam, for instance, the youngest of the world's major religions, originated 1,300 years ago and is not a strong supporter of the vegetarian ideal. Christianity, 2,000 years old, offers a bit more evidence for the practicality of the meatless way of life. And Judaism, about 4,000 years old, has a large tradition of vegetarianism. One of the most ancient religions known, Hinduism, is a strong supporter of vegetarian principles. Buddhism and Jainism, while only some 2,500 years old, are essentially Hindu heterodoxies, and so fully share the vegetarian principles upheld by their parent religion, often to a much greater degree.

There are exceptions to this rule. Some modern denominations do indeed promulgate vegetarianism. Seventh-Day Adventists, Quakers and Mormons, for example, have a meatless contingent. And while Sufis are an exception among the Muslims, the Baha'i Faith also endorses vegetarianism (although meat-products are not strictly forbidden). These are exceptions, however, and in general the above rule holds true: the older the religion, the closer to vegetarianism.

Now, to many, the fact that the more ancient religious traditions uphold the vegetarian ideal is proof that vegetarianism is a dated concept, a primitive ideal maintained by superstition or ignorance. To others, the antiquity of vegetarianism stands as a major indication of its primacy in religious thought, before the purity of faith and doctrine was subjected to later revisions, interpretations, or accommodations.

The earliest forms of religious expression fully accept vegetarianism—if not always in practice then at least in scriptural principle. Scripture is here defined as those literary works on which a religion was originally founded, as opposed to later interpretive writings. Any explanation of scriptural teaching—including my own—is in one sense "interpretive." However, since scriptures are held sacred by their respective followers, they should be understood as they were originally intended. This book therefore endeavors to remain as close to original intent as possible by referring to primary sources and literal translations. One may compare and verify, for example, all Bible passages throughout this work by referring to Reuben Alcalay's *Complete Hebrew-English-Dictionary* for the Old Testament, and to *Nestle's Interlinear Greek-English New Testament.*

Of course, most people do not read their scriptures this way. The tendency is for believers to accept whatever edition or translation of original scripture their church happens to favor at any particular time. And most such popular editions are not translated rigorously or with a view toward understanding the original meaning of the texts. The philosophical and theological problem with this, however, is considerable. The value of unaltered scripture is analogous to that of a computer instruction manual. It goes without saying that such a complicated apparatus as a computer needs an instruction booklet for proper operation. In the complex universe we inhabit, scriptures act like instruction manuals, guiding us through the intricacies of universal law and function. Further, where a man-made instruction manual may be imperfect and subject to revision, God's law books, by definition, are absolute and eternal, with few differences according to time, place and circumstance. Therefore, if it can be shown that one of the original intents of the world's major religious scriptures was to encourage a meatless diet, then this book contends that any person who even nominally claims to adhere to a particular faith cannot morally justify eating meat.

The Scientific Perspective

Before any discussion of the religious and moral rationale for vegetarianism, an examination of the scientific reasons for avoiding flesh as a food source should be given. Modern medicine offers ample evidence of the dangers of meat-eating. Cancer and heart disease are nearly epidemic in nations with a high per capita consumption of meat, while they rarely occur in societies where little meat is consumed. There is also considerable scientific evidence that the teeth, jaws, and the long, convoluted intestinal canal in humans are not naturally suited to a diet containing meat. The value of this evidence in the present context is that vegetarianism on purely abstract or philosophical grounds rarely lasts. Without an awareness of the dietary facts, even the most ardent religionists are apt to adopt a meat-oriented diet. On the other hand, it would be incomplete to adhere to a meatless diet without understanding its deeper meaning for humanity.

As a side issue, it should be noted that a true religionist would find it difficult to tolerate the suffering inflicted upon animals in the slaughterhouse. For example, steers are routinely castrated to make them more docile. Castration also promotes a fattier, more profitable animal. Castration can be done radically, all at once, or over a longer period of time with a ring-like instrument, causing the testicles to gradually fall away. And although drugs are an integral part of today's agriculture, anesthetics are rarely used for this procedure, especially in the United States. In fact, cruelty is a regular occurrence at stockyards. Sick and crippled farm animals, called "downers," often lie suffering for days until dragged by chain to slaughter. The downer phenomenon would drastically be reduced if all stockyards refused to allow ranchers to make any money on them. (Slaughter of a living creature affords a rancher a better price than "dead-on-arrival" meat.) But this will never happen.

Moreover, such torture exists for all "food" animals, no matter what the species. For example, it is not uncommon in most factory hen-houses for several hens to be squeezed into a rather small, 12"x18" cage. This causes unbearable suffering for them, which causes them to go crazy. At this point, it is standard procedure for poultry producers to "de-beak" chicks with hot-knife machines, something that is even more painful than being stuffed in the same hen-house for long periods. Despite the pain, however, de-beaking is likely to continue, for it is the only reliable method, say the factory farmers, to stop the tortured birds from pecking each other to death.

Furthermore, in egg factories throughout the country, male chicks are weeded out and disposed of by "chick-pullers." Daily, over 500,000 of these chicks are stuffed en masse into plastic bags, where they are suffocated and crushed. Or, sometimes, they are ground up while still alive to be fed to livestock or used as fertilizer. Such horrors are not uncommon, but the public is just now becoming aware of these things. As science and technology move forward, let us hope that more humane treatment of animals is on the horizon, and that education will afford us a more sensible diet, one in which other living creatures need not sacrifice their lives for our arbitrary culinary preferences.

In the remaining portion of the introduction, we shall outline a few of the secular, practical reasons for the vegetarian way of life, and then we will begin to explore the various world religions, to see what they teach in regard to the meatless diet and man's treatment of animals.

The Protein Myth

Fear of protein deficiency is why many people never adopt a vegetarian diet. "Can one get good quality protein—and all one needs—from a non-meat diet?" they ask. Before answering this question, let us first define protein.

In 1838, a Dutch chemist, Gerrit Jan Mulder, isolated a substance containing nitrogen, carbon, hydrogen, oxygen and other trace elements. He showed this chemical compound to be the basis of all life, and he named it protein, meaning "first rank." It has been subsequently proven that protein is biologically essential: every living organism must ingest a certain amount of it to survive. This, it was found, is due to the fact that proteins are composed of amino acids, the "building blocks" of life.

Plants can synthesize amino acids from air, earth and water, but animals are dependent on plants for protein, either directly by eating plants or indirectly by eating an animal which has eaten and metabolized plants. Only the vegetable kingdom is capable of producing protein. Thus, humans have the option of obtaining it directly and with great efficiency from plants, or indirectly and at great expense, both financially and in terms of resources consumed, from animal flesh. (One reason for the latter's higher cost is that the animal has been forced to eat a tremendous amount of vegetable proteins in order to reach slaughter weight.)

There are thus no amino acids in flesh that animals do not derive from plants, or that humans cannot also derive from plants. Moreover, eating foods from the plant kingdom has the added advantage of combining amino acids with other substances that are essential to the proper utilization of protein: carbohydrates, vitamins, minerals, enzymes, hormones, chlorophyll, and other elements that only plants can supply.

However, vegetarians should know the theory of food-combining, which some natural biologists say is essential if one wishes to obtain "complete" proteins. This concept, better known as "protein complementary," was popularized by Frances Moore Lappe in her best-selling book, *Diet for a Small Planet*, where she explains that complementary proteins are usually put together as a matter of course in a balanced vegetarian diet. If we eat peanut butter, for example, we smear it on some bread; this is how one generally eats peanut butter. If we use whole grain bread, we would have a generous amount of protein. Here is how this works.

When we eat, the body breaks the protein down into its constituent amino acids. These are either utilized individually or reassembled into new proteins needed by the body. There are twenty-two known amino acids. Fourteen are "non-essential" and eight are "essential." ("Essential" here simply means that we cannot manufacture them naturally within the body and must get them from our food.)

The essential amino acids are leucine, isoleucine, valine, lysine, tryptophan, threonine, methionine and phenylalanine. All of these must appear, according to Lappe, during the day in the right proportions to have a well-balanced diet. For this reason, up to the mid-1950s meat was considered an excellent source of protein: it has all eight essential amino acids in the proper proportions. Nonetheless, nutritionists now agree that many vegetarian foods are equal to, if not better than, meat in terms of protein content, for these foods contain all eight amino acids as well.

In general, the rule for producing high-protein vegetarian dishes is to combine grains (breads, pasta, etc.) with legumes (soybeans, lentils, peanuts, etc.) at the same meal—as is done with the previously mentioned peanut butter sandwich. Nuts and seeds combined with legumes or even with cereals also provide a high-protein diet. If milk products are included in the diet, there is even less chance of a protein problem, for milk also contains all of the essential amino acids. It has also been determined that many green, leafy vegetables and even potatoes have a considerable amount of complete protein. And an eight-ounce glass of carrot juice has the same quality and amount of protein as an egg.

Dr. John A. McDougall, Assistant Clinical Professor at the University of Hawaii Medical School and Medical Director of the Lifestyle and Nutrition Program at St. Helena Hospital in Deer Park, California, says that protein complementary is unnecessary.[1] He claims there is more than enough protein in individual vegetarian foods. Other authorities agree with him,[2] and Lappe's concept of complementary protein, while strongly supported by nutritional experts in its day, has been challenged. Nonetheless, whether one feels the need to combine foods or is equally comfortable without food combination, there is ample evidence that vegetarianism is simple, healthful, and capable of supplying the required amounts of protein.

In 1954 a group of scientists at Harvard University conducted a study and found that when a variety of vegetables, grains and dairy products were eaten together, the combination produced more than adequate supplies of daily protein.[3] Their report concluded that it was actually quite difficult to eat a varied vegetarian diet that would not exceed protein requirements for the human body. More recently, in 1972, Dr. F. Stare at Harvard conducted his own study of protein intake among vegetarians. His findings were startling: the majority of subjects were consuming twice their minimum daily protein requirement.[4] Similar studies were conducted by the late Dr. Paavo Airola, one of the twentieth century's leading authorities on nutrition and natural biology. His findings conclusively proved that vegetarians need not have a protein problem and that protein was as easily available to them as to the meat-eater.[5]

It is the current position of the American Dietetic Association that vegetarian diets are healthful and nutritionally adequate when appropriately planned. This was confirmed, with a lengthy report, in the November 1993 issue of their journal. Moreover, this view is now supported by the "Dietary Guidelines for Americans," a statement representing current federal policy on the role of dietary factors in health promotion and disease prevention. These Guidelines were issued by the Department of Agriculture (USDA) and Health and Human Services—both very mainstream and conservative organizations—first in 1980, and then in 1985 and 1990. The fourth edition has recently been released, and, for the first time ever, the health recommendations mention vegetarianism directly: "Some Americans eat vegetarian diets for reasons of culture, belief, or health. Most vegetarians eat dairy products and eggs and, as a group, these lacto-ovo-vegetarians enjoy excellent health. Vegetarian diets are consistent with the Dietary Guidelines and can meet Recommended Dietary Allowances for nutrients. Protein is not limiting in vegetarian diets as long as the variety and amounts of foods consumed are adequate." This report was issued by the Dietary Guidelines Advisory Committee on the Dietary Guidelines for Americans in September, 1995, and is a great breakthrough for the vegetarian way of life.

Meat-Eating and World Hunger

Consider the following statistics. One thousand acres of soybeans yield 1,124 pounds of usable protein. One thousand acres of rice yield 938 pounds of usable protein. One thousand acres of corn yield 1,009 pounds of usable protein. One thousand acres of wheat yield 1,043 pounds of usable protein. Now consider this: one thousand acres of soybeans, corn, rice or wheat, *when fed to a steer*, will yield only about 125 pounds of usable protein.[6] These and other findings point to a disturbing conclusion: meat-eating is directly related to world hunger.

Some nutritionists, environmentalists and politicians have pointed out that if the United States were to feed that same grain and soy supply to the poor and starving people of the world as is fed to livestock, we could wipe out starvation and its corollary horrors.[7] In fact, Harvard nutritionist Jean Mayer estimates that reducing meat production by just ten percent would release enough grain to feed sixty million people.[8] It is a matter of record: in terms of land, water and resources, meat is the most expensive and inefficient "food" anyone can eat. Only about ten percent of the protein and calories we feed to livestock is returned in the meat those animals provide. In addition, hundreds of thousands of acres of arable land are occupied in raising livestock for food. One acre used to raise a steer provides only about one pound of protein. That same one acre planted with soybeans will produce seventeen pounds of protein.[9] In short, raising animals for food is a tremendous waste of the world's resources.

In addition to the loss of farmland, it is estimated that raising livestock consumes eight times more water than growing vegetables, soy or grains, for the cattle must drink and the crops that feed them must be watered. In summary, millions will continue to die of thirst or starvation, while a privileged few consume vast amounts of protein, wasting land and water in the process. Ironically, this same meat is their own body's worst enemy.

It is now known, too, that meat-eating threatens our environment. For example, methane is one of the four greenhouse gases that contributes to the environmental trend known as global warming. The 1.3 billion cattle in the world produce one-fifth of all the methane emitted into the atmosphere. According to a most informative article in the January 15, 1993 edition of *The Washington Spectator*, most of this cattle-raising is specifically done to provide meat for the kitchen table. If this were avoided, says the article, it would be a major step toward rectifying the problem of global warming. Moreover, the world's invaluable rain forests tend to be victimized by the lumber and meat industries. Much of Central America was transformed into a giant pasture to provide cheap beef for North America, while in South America the Amazon rain forests were cleared and burned to make room for cattle grazing, largely to supply the beef needs of England and Europe. These ideas are developed by Jeremy Rifkin in his excellent book, *Beyond Beef.* Rifkin makes a clear connection between meat-eating and the degradation of the environment, explaining that the earth will not support us in our avarice and ignorance. Rather, he says, quoting Gandhi, "The earth can supply everything for man's need, but not for his greed."

Clearly, our greed is quickly depleting the earth. Recent marginal growth in animal protein consumption in increasingly affluent and developing countries has led to huge increases in the need for feed grains. For example, in 1995, China went—virtually overnight—from being an exporter to an importer of grain. This points to a problem that will only get worse: world shortages are predicted as both populations and meat consumption increase simultaneously—a combination that is simply not sustainable. In a recent *BusinessWeek* article (February 12, 1996), it was reported that, according to the Worldwatch Institute, the world "may have crossed a threshold where even the best efforts of governments to build stocks may not be enough." Mass vegetarianism may be the only answer, but, of course, it is not likely.

Meat-Eating and Poor Health

When an animal is slaughtered, the waste products normally taken away by the animal's bloodstream are retained in the decaying flesh. Meat-eaters absorb into their own bodies the toxic wastes that would otherwise have been expelled from the animal's body as urine. Dr. Owen S. Parrett, in his paper "Why I Don't Eat Meat," notes that when steak is boiled, waste appears as a soluble extract in the form of beef tea—which closely resembles urine when chemically analyzed.[10]

Meat in industrialized nations that practice intensive agriculture is also loaded with preservatives: DDT, arsenic (used in cattle feed as a growth stimulant), sodium sulfate (used to give meat that "fresh" red color) and DES, a synthetic hormone that is a known carcinogen.[11] In fact, meat products include many agents that are either carcinogenic or metastasizers of cancer. For instance, in just over two pounds of charcoal-broiled steak, there is as much benzopyrene as contained in the smoke from 600 cigarettes![12] As the famous Christian theologian and practicing vegetarian, Dr. J. H. Kellogg, once remarked when he sat down to a colorful vegetarian dinner, "It's nice to eat a meal and not have to worry about what your food may have died of."[13]

Perhaps the single most compelling argument for a non-meat diet, at least as far as personal health goes, is the undeniable and well-documented correlation between meat-eating and heart disease. In America, the highest meat-consuming nation in the world, one person out of every two will die of heart or related vascular diseases. These diseases are practically nonexistent in cultures where meat consumption is low. *The Journal of the American Medical Association* reported in 1961 that a "vegetarian diet can prevent ninety to ninety-seven percent of heart disease."[14] Since a non-meat diet lessens cholesterol intake, there is less chance of fat build-up and thus death from a stroke or a heart attack; the condition known as arteriosclerosis is virtually unknown in the vegetarian world. According to the *Encyclopedia Britannica,* "Protein obtained from nuts, pulses, grains, and even dairy products is said to be relatively pure compared with beef—which has a fifty-six percent impure water content."[15] Such impurity affects not only the heart, but the whole human organism.

Meat-eating is killing us. According to *Eat Right, Live Longer* (1995), by Neal Barnard, M.D., "Vegetarian diets are much better than diets including even modest amounts of animal products. The National Cancer Institute adopted a Five-a-Day program, encouraging Americans to consume five servings of vegetables and fruits every day. That is a great start, but we also need a 'Zero-a-Day' program to eliminate meats and dairy products." Actually, the connection between cancer and meat-eating is now well-known, and John Robbins, in his popular book, *Diet for a New America,* cites prominent authorities when he writes, "Meat-centered diets are linked to many types of cancer, most notably cancer of the colon, breast, cervix, uterus, ovary, prostate, and lung." Conversely, diets rich in the Four New Food Groups—whole grains, vegetable, fruits, and legumes, established in 1991 by the Physicians Committee for Responsible Medicine, and completely out-moding the prior four food groups, namely, meat, dairy, grains, and fruits and vegetables (lumped together as one category!)—are said to help prevent cancer. This is fully documented in Neal Barnard's excellent work, *Food for Life.*

According to Dr. T. Colin Campbell, one of the key researchers involved with "The China Study" (which is the largest study of diet and health ever conducted), "In the next ten to fifteen years, one of the things you're bound to hear is that animal protein...is one of the most toxic nutrients of all..." He added that risk for disease goes up dramatically when even a little animal protein is added to the diet. This is understandable when one considers that meat contains approximately fourteen times more pesticides than plant foods. And so, after some time, the human body just refuses to deal with these toxins, giving way to disease and, finally, death.

The National Heart, Lung and Blood Institute estimates that cardiovascular diseases were responsible for 954,000 deaths (42% of all deaths) in 1993. They further estimate that the total direct cost to sufferers added up to about $126.4 billion. Seventy-two percent of the deaths were due to atherosclerosis (hardening of the arteries), a disease strongly linked to meat-eating. Such findings are becoming well-known: a recent article in the *New York Times* (November 21, 1995) gave elaborate evidence of the high price we are paying for health problems associated with meat-eating—the Physicians Committee for Responsible Medicine, a group of 3,000 physicians, estimated the annual health care costs directly resulting from the nation's meat-centered diet to be between $23.6 billion and $61.4 billion (comparable to similar health cost estimates associated with cigarette smoking). We are indeed paying a high price for meat-eating, both in terms of our own health and for hospital bills.

And then there is Bovine Spongiform Encephalopathy (BSE), also known as "Mad Cow Disease." This is a condition in which cows display unsightly mental torture and then die—it is a terminal neuro-degenerative cattle disease caused by toxic, virulent and mysterious infectious proteins called *prions*. An outbreak in England had by early 1996 stricken some 160,000 cows. Evidence pointed to the British practice of mixing the remains of sheep, including their brains and bones, into cows' feed as the cause of the outbreak. This apparent species-to-species inoculation is what makes all forms of spongiform encephalopathy (known to affect other mammals as well) so disturbing. What's more, it is now theorized that cow-eating humans may be the next victims of this horrible disease. Recent reports suggest that a certain strain of Creutzfeldt-Jacob Disease (CJD) may be the human variant of spongiform encephalopathy. Grim but conservative predictions tell of up to 500,000 Britons a year dying of this disease due to their past consumption of BSE-infected cows. *Prion*-based diseases often have incubation periods that take decades, much like AIDS, so we are only beginning to see the long-term consequences of this outbreak. Meanwhile, reports of an American strain are starting to appear in medical journals—if this doesn't give meat-eaters food for thought, nothing will.

The human body is a complex machine. Like all machines, some fuels are more appropriate than others to keep it running smoothly. The record shows that meat is a very inefficient fuel for the human machine, one that eventually exacts a severe toll. Eskimos, for example, who live primarily on meat and fish, age rapidly. Their average life span rarely exceeds thirty years. The Kirgese, an Eastern Russian people that at one time lived chiefly on meat, rarely survived past the age of forty. On the other hand, there are tribes such as the Hunza, who live in the Himalayan Mountains, or groups like the Seventh-Day Adventists, a primarily vegetarian Christian group, who tend to live between eighty and 100 years. Researchers cite vegetarianism as the reason for their excellent health and longevity. The Maya Indians of Yucatan and the Yemenite tribe of Semitic origin are also known for their excellent health, and a low meat or in some cases 100 percent vegetarian diet is again cited as the main contributory factor.

Anatomical Evidence

When eating meat, human beings disguise it in a variety of ways, using ketchup, sauces and gravies. They age it, tenderize it, fry it, boil it, and transform it in a thousand styles. Why the charade? Why all the effort to avoid eating meat raw, as all true carnivorous animals do? Many nutritionists, biologists and physiologists offer convincing evidence that humans are in fact not meant to eat flesh. They propose that people are not physiologically suited to a carnivorous diet and that the reason they disguise it is that it is an unnatural food.

Physiologically, people are more akin to plant-eaters, foragers and grazers, such as monkeys, elephants and cows, than to carnivora, such as dogs, tigers and leopards.[16] For example, carnivora do not sweat through their skin; body heat is controlled by rapid breathing and extrusion of the tongue. Vegetarian animals, on the other hand, have sweat pores for heat control and the elimination of impurities. Carnivora have long teeth and claws for holding and killing prey; vegetarian animals have short teeth and no claws. The saliva of carnivora contains no ptyalin and cannot predigest starches; that of vegetarian animals contains ptyalin for the predigestion of starches. Flesh-eating animals secrete large quantities of hydrochloric acid to help dissolve bones; vegetarian animals secrete little hydrochloric acid. The jaws of carnivora only open in an up-and-down motion; those of vegetarian animals also move sideways for additional kinds of chewing. Carnivora must lap liquids (like a cat); vegetarian animals take liquids in by suction through the teeth. There are many such comparisons, and in each case humans fit the vegetarian physiognomy.[17] From a strictly physiological perspective, then, there are strong arguments that humans are not suited to a fleshy diet.

And speaking of physiognomy, there is a related question: what about plant bodies? Are they designed to be eaten? Do they not feel pain? Are they not living, breathing creatures that are worthy of our compassion? "If all life is sacred," some people challenge, "then why do you consider it appropriate to eat plants?" People who raise such questions often think of vegetarianism as a type of hypocrisy.

This mode of questioning was crystallized for me in 1984, when *The Philadelphia Inquirer Magazine* ran an editorial, asking, "Is it not hypocritical to avoid eating animals but to continue eating plants? Both are living things!" The editor of the *Inquirer* asked this question as a reaction to an essay by William Ecenbarger, in that same issue, which eloquently articulated the concerns of the animal rights movement. Ecenbarger explained, using impressive documentation, that it is only due to ignorance and greed that we continue to abuse animals—it is nothing more than a form of "speciesism," he said. He showed how the cause of animal rights is cut from the same moral cloth as other crusades against injustice—the struggle against racism and sexism, for example. (An elaborate treatment of these issues can be seen in Carol Adams' excellent book *The Sexual Politics of Meat: A Feminist-Vegetarian Critical Theory.*) Perhaps the strongest argument against speciesism is summed up in a quote from the British philosopher Jeremy Bentham (1748-1832), who wrote in his now famous *Principles of Morals and Legislation*: "The question is not, Can they reason? nor, Can they think? but, Can they suffer? The answer, of course, is an unequivocal 'Yes, animals certainly *can* suffer.' Just as we can suffer, so can they." Therefore, say animal rightists, we should logically extend our sense of ethics to include animals.

This is reasonable enough. But David R. Boldt, who wrote the editorial mentioned above, raised what seems to be an equally reasonable objection: "My own excuse for eating meat is that plants, research has shown, have feelings, just like animals. Why choose between them? Before considering the fate of the steer, imagine the dread and horror that spreads across a wheat field when the thresher starts its work."

Boldt's challenge is misleading, if also held by many. He refers to documentation that plants have feelings—and while even the work of Jagdish Chandra Bhosh, from the nineteenth century, will attest to the fact that plants do indeed have feelings, such rudimentary sensations are clearly distinguishable from the pain of a steer going to slaughter. We all know this. Our stomachs react considerably less if we observe the threshing of a wheat field than if we observe the grisly work in a slaughterhouse. Moreover, as Keith Akers writes in *The Vegetarian Sourcebook*, "Finding an ethically significant line between plants and animals...is not particularly difficult. Plants have no evolutionary need to feel pain, and completely lack a central nervous system. Nature does not create pain gratuitously, but only when it enables the organism to survive. Animals, being mobile, would benefit from having a sense of pain; plants would not."

Clearly, if one does not want to become a fruitarian, waiting only for certain fruits to naturally drop from a tree, vegetarianism is a practical alternative. And even if one believes that plants have feelings much like humans and animals (despite evidence to the contrary), it still does not follow that vegetarianism is hypocritical: if plants can suffer, but we need to eat them to survive, it makes sense to eat as few as possible. In other words, if we *have to* eat plants, a fact upon which all biologists and nutritionists agree, we ought to destroy as few plants as possible. But by raising and eating an animal for food, many more plants are destroyed indirectly by the animal we eat than if we merely ate the plants directly. So vegetarianism causes the least amount of harm to sentient beings, and one who thinks deeply about all of the issues involved will surely see the sense of the vegetarian alternative.

Spiritual Vegetarianism

Even if the scientific facts didn't tally, there are compelling spiritual reasons for vegetarianism. Consider, for instance, that the word "spiritual" comes from the Latin *spiritus*, meaning "breath," "vigor," or "life." The word "vegetarian" comes from the Greek *vegetas*, or "full of the breath of life." Even the etymology of the two words affirms their interrelation.

Along these same lines, it may be worthwhile to note that the words "carnal" and "carnivorous" come from the same root, which is the Latin *carnis*, meaning "flesh." All religious scriptures suggest that votaries avoid carnality, and in the biblical tradition that which is "carnal" belongs distinctly to the world of flesh as opposed to spirit.

Parenthetically, while etymology is an interesting science, this author is aware of its limitations and/or misapplication. Well-meaning vegetarians have for too long attacked the meat industry's "word games," claiming that moneymakers in the industry tend to disguise animal products with innocuous pseudo names: pig/pork, calf/veal, cow/beef, sheep/mutton, and so on. On this score, the meat industry is thoroughly innocent. The way it happened is something like this: in mediaeval England, the peasants were Anglo-Saxon but the aristocracy was Norman-French. Although the peasants looked after the animals, it was mainly the aristocracy who ate the meat. Be that as it may, the peasants referred to the animals by their Anglo-Saxon names—pig, calf, sheep, and so on, but the aristocracy—the meat-eaters themselves—called the same animals in French, i.e., *porc* (pig), *veau* (calf), *boeuf* (ox or bullock), *mouton* (sheep). These words were eventually Anglicized, but the distinction between these animals and the meat they become has remained standard in every English-speaking country of the world. As a sort of further proof in this direction, one might note that animals which were not commonly eaten by the Norman-French aristocracy, e.g., chicken, turkey, rabbit, etc., have the same name for the animal as for that of the meat that comes from them.

The connection between vegetarianism and religion, however, goes beyond semantics and ultimately touches upon the very essence of religious truth. For instance, it is often reasonably postulated that God naturally loves His works, which include not only humans but all other species of life. If this basic tenet is accepted, *then no living entity is beyond the scope of God's compassion,* and *no* unnecessary killing would be approved. This theological basis for vegetarianism is especially prominent in Hinduism. In the West, it was upheld by the early Jews and even the ancient Greeks, such as Diogenes, Pythagoras, Socrates and Plato, who termed vegetarianism *antikreophagy,* or "anti-flesh-eating."

God's compassion and love for His creation denote another, often overlooked, reason for vegetarianism. With the mounting scientific evidence that a meatless diet offers a more healthful life, and that eating flesh shortens one's lifespan, reason dictates that God would choose a vegetarian diet for His children. Why would one who loves His creation desire its quick demise? Clearly, He would not. In fact, He would take great pains to insure its longevity. Accordingly, God tries in the scriptures, time and again, to assure His children that vegetarianism is the best possible diet for them. Mainstream religions—particularly in the West—have minimized this idea. Nonetheless, we will show that universal religious thought promotes universal compassion, and condemns the opposite—the unnecessary slaughter of living beings—as fundamentally irreligious.

REFERENCES

1. John and Mary McDougall, "The Latest Thinking On Protein," *Vegetarian Times,* March 1986, No. 103, p. 26.
2. John A. Scharffenberg, *Problems With Meat* (CA, Woodbridge Press, 1982), pp. 85-86.
3. M. G. Hardinge and F. J. Stare, "Nutritional Studies of Vegetarians," *American Journal of Clinical Nutrition,* 2:73, 1954, p. 76.
4. Committee on Nutritional Misinformation, National Academy of Sciences, "Can a Vegetarian Be Well Nourished?," *Journal of the American Medical Association,* Vol. 233, No. 8, (August 25, 1975) p. 898.
5. Paavo Airola, *Are You Confused?* (Arizona, Health Plus Pub., 1971), pp. 32-33.
6. Philip Handler, "Science, Food and Man's Future," *Borden Review of Nutrition Research,* Vol. 31, No. 1, January-March, 1971, p. 9.
7. Barbara Parham, *What's Wrong with Eating Meat?* (Colorado, Ananda Marg Pub., 1979), p. 38.
8. Jean Mayer, Cited by the U.S. Senate Select Committee on Nutrition and Human Needs, *Dietary Goals for the U.S.* (Washington, DC, February, 1977), p. 44.
9. Francis Moore Lappe, *Diet for a Small Planet* (New York, Ballantine Books, 1975, reprint 1982), pp. 69-71.
10. Owen S. Parrett, *Diseases of Food Animals* (Washington, DC, Review and Herald Pub., 1974), pp. 26-27.
11. Raymond H. Woolsey, *Meat on the Menu: Who Needs It?* (Washington, DC, Review and Herald Pub., 1974), pp. 40-50.
12. W. Lijinsky and P. Shubik, "Benzo(a)pyrene and other polynuclear hydrocarbons in charcoal-broiled meat," *Science,* 145:53, 55, 1964.
13. J. H. Kellogg, *The Natural Diet of Man* (Michigan, Modern Medicine Pub., 1923; reprint, N.J., The Edenite Society, 1979), pp. 67-68.
14. W. A. Thomas, editor, "Diet and Stress in Vascular Disease," *Journal of the American Medical Association,* 176:9, June 3, 1961, p. 806.
15. Barbara Parham, *op. cit.,* p. 15.
16. G. S. Huntington, *The Anatomy of the Human Peritoneum and Abdominal Cavity* (New York, Lea Brothers, 1903), pp. 189-199.
17. W. S. Collens and G. B. Dobkin, "Phylogenetic aspects of the cause of human atherosclerotic disease," *Circulation,* Suppl. 11, 32:7, October, 1965.

CHRISTIANITY
Chapter 1

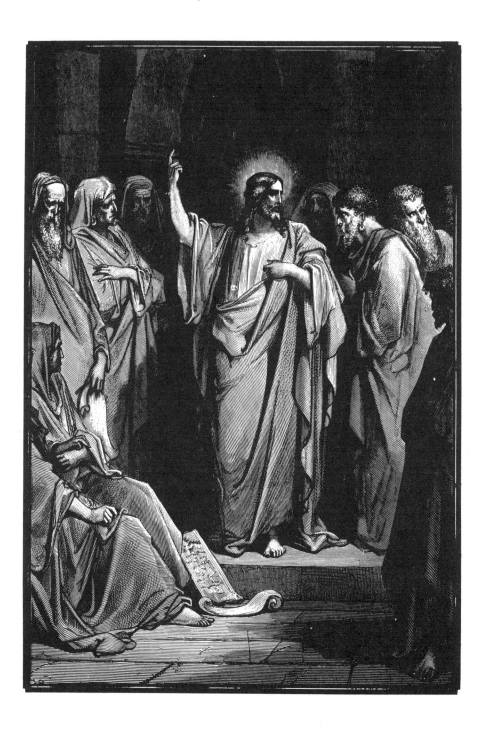

CHRISTIANITY

*"Take care not to destroy God's work for the
sake of something to eat."*

—Romans 14:20

Although the New Testament focuses almost exclusively on Jesus, little is known about his diet. There were, however, many early Christians and chroniclers of Christian tradition who did support vegetarianism, including such luminaries as St. Jerome, Tertullian, St. John Chrysostom, St. Benedict, Clement, Eusebius, Pliny, Papias, Cyprian, Pantaenus and John Wesley, to name a few. Like Jesus and the Biblical prophets, they taught, by their words and deeds, that mercy and compassion should extend to all creatures—a definition far broader than that held by most Christians today.

The Bible—including the Old Testament, since Christianity has its origins in Judaism—is the best place to begin a study of Christianity and vegetarianism. The Old Testament deals mainly with the Jews receiving the laws of God and later being punished by God for breaking them. The New Testament shows Jesus bestowing God's forgiveness on the truly repentant, stressing that the first and foremost commandment is to love God with all one's heart, mind and soul.

Still, history shows that this commandment was rarely followed, and the Old Testament records that God would often grant a concession and relax certain laws, trying to encourage the lawbreakers to partially follow His commands and thus gradually develop their love for Him. But the original dietary law reveals God's preference:

19

> And behold, I have given you every herb-bearing seed, which is upon the face of all the earth, and every tree, in which is the fruit of a tree-yielding seed—to you it shall be for food....And God saw everything He had made, and behold, it was very good...(Genesis, 1:29, 31)

If God saw His original dietary law as "very good," why did He later give so many instructions for eating flesh? According to Deuteronomy, it was out of compassion for the "lustful Israelites":

> When the Lord thy God shall enlarge thy border, as He hath promised thee, and thou shalt say, "I will eat flesh," because thy soul longeth to eat flesh; thou mayest eat flesh, or whatsoever thy soul lusteth after. (Deut. 12:20)

Some people argue that in Genesis 9:3 the Bible allows humans to eat meat: "Every moving thing that lives shall be food for you." This, however, is in the account of the great flood, when Noah was provided with an expedient in a crisis. As all vegetation was destroyed, God indeed gave Noah a *concession*—not a commandment—to eat meat. But the ideal diet, it should be remembered, was given earlier, and God said it was "very good." That phrase was never used to describe later diets containing meat.

In fact, in the very next verse, Genesis 9:4, after having given permission to eat every moving thing, God reminds us once again that we should ideally not eat flesh, or at least the blood: "But you should not eat flesh with its life, that is, its blood." And further, the next verse clearly states that the people who kill the animals will, in turn, be killed by those very same creatures: "And your life will I seek, at the hand of every creature you slay..."[1]

Actually, some scholars observe that when Noah was given the right to eat every moving thing, the exact Greek word used in the Septuagint was *herpeton*, which literally means "reptile."[2] Thus, when no other food was available, God gave him permission to eat crustaceans and mollusks, such as clams, abalone, lobsters and snails. This, in fact, is actually more consistent with Genesis 9:4, which prohibits Noah from eating animals with blood (he was only allowed cold-blooded creatures)—and again, only temporarily as a concession.

According to author Joseph Benson, "It ought to be observed that the prohibition of eating blood, given to Noah and all his posterity, and repeated to the Israelites...has never been revoked, but, on the contrary, it has been confirmed under the New Testament, Acts XV; it is, thereby, a perpetual obligation."[3]

The Christian theologian Etienne de Courcelles (1586-1659) was convinced that the Apostles had thus discouraged at least the eating of blood, if not meat altogether: "Although some of our brothers would reckon it a crime to shed human blood, they did not think the same about eating animal [blood]. The Apostles, by their decree, wished to remedy the ignorance of these persons."[4]

There were many who spoke out in this regard, and history relates that when the early Christians were accused of eating children, a woman named Biblis (A.D. 177) protested: "How would such men eat children, when they are not even allowed to eat the blood of irrational animals?"[5]

Later, during the Trullan council held at Constantinople in A.D. 692, the following rule was established: "The eating of the blood of animals is forbidden in holy scripture. A cleric who partakes of blood is to be punished by deposition, a layman with excommunication."[6]

Returning to Christian roots and the tradition of the Old Testament for a moment, another prohibition against the eating of blood appears in Leviticus 7:26, which says, "Moreover, ye shall eat no manner of blood, whether it be of fowl or of beast, in any of your dwellings." Many interpret this as a commandment to drain the meat of blood and then to eat it anyway (see chapter on Judaism). There is one other instance in the *Five Books of Moses* when God, as a temporary concession, allowed the Israelites to eat meat, but again this was in dire circumstances. After fleeing Egypt, the Israelites wandered forty years in the wilderness. God provided food in the form of *manna* ("the staff of life"), a miraculous vegetarian substance that provided every life-sustaining element needed. But the Israelites tired of *manna*, the Bible tells us, so God arranged to give the children of Israel meat in the form of quail. Why quail? Was there some hidden teaching God was trying to convey?

Numbers 11:18-34 reveals the answer. In verse 20, God tells them to "eat flesh until it comes out of your nostrils and it becomes loathsome to you..." Verse 33 tells us that "before the flesh was even between their teeth, a great plague struck them down." In effect, they were allowed the change in diet, but God was clearly dissatisfied with their choice. The burial places of those Israelites, incidentally, have traditionally been referred to as "the graves of lust" because they desired something they did not need: meat.

Centuries later, when the small Jewish sect called "Christianity" came into being, it adopted several of the attitudes and traditions of its parent faith, including meat-eating. But there have been some very important exceptions, both in Judaism and Christianity. And the vegetarian tradition played a significant role in the lives of the early Christians.

Christian Vegetarians

Some historical documents claim that the twelve Apostles and even Judas' replacement, Matthias, were vegetarians, and that the early Christians abstained from meat-eating on the grounds of purity and mercy. For example, St. John Chrysostom (A.D. 345-407), one of the most outstanding Christian literary advocates of his time, wrote, "We, the Christian leaders, practice abstinence from the flesh of animals to subdue our bodies...the unnatural eating of flesh-meat is polluting."[7]

Clement of Alexandria (A.D. 160-240), an early church academician, obviously had great influence on Chrysostom, for nearly 100 years before, he had written: "But those who bend around inflammatory tables, nourishing their own diseases, are ruled by a most lickerish demon, whom I shall not blush to call belly-demon, and the worst of all demons...It is far better to be happy than to have our bodies act as graveyards for animals. Accordingly, the Apostle Matthew partook of seeds, nuts and vegetables, without flesh."[8]

The *Clementine Homilies*, also written in the second century, is said to be based on the preaching of St. Peter and is considered one of the earliest Christian texts, barring only the Bible. *Homily XII* boldly declares, "The unnatural eating of flesh-meats is as polluting as the heathen worship of devils, with its sacrifices and its impure feasts, through participation in which a man becomes a fellow eater with devils." Who are we to argue with St. Peter?

Further, there is some scholarly debate about St. Paul's dietary practices, despite the cavalier attitude about diet found in his writings. Acts 24:5 speaks of Paul as being from the Nazarene sect—a sect which followed Essene principles, including vegetarianism. And according to Dr. Edgar Goodspeed, in his book *History of Early Christianity*, there was once an "Acts of Thomas" used by early Christian sects. This document describes St. Thomas as abstaining from flesh-foods as well. Meanwhile, we learn from the distinguished Church father Eusebius (A.D. 264-349), in his quotation of Hegesippus (c. A.D. 160), that James, accepted by many as the brother of Christ, also refrained from eating the flesh of animals.[9]

Still, history relates that organized Christendom gradually moved away from its vegetarian roots. Although the early Christian fathers adhered to a meatless regimen, more recently, the Roman Catholic Church had ruled that practicing Catholics at least observe certain fast days and abstain from eating meat on Fridays (in remembrance of the sacrificial death of Christ). Even this stricture was compromised, however, when, in 1966, the U.S. Catholic Conference determined that Catholics need only abstain from eating meat on the Fridays of Lent.

Many early Christian groups supported the meatless way of life. In fact, the writings of the early Church indicate that meat-eating was not officially allowed until the fourth century, when the Emperor Constantine decided that his version of Christianity would be the version for everyone. A meat-eating interpretation of the Bible became the official creed of the Roman Empire, and vegetarian Christians had to practice in secret or risk being put to death for heresy. It is said that Constantine used to pour molten lead down their throats if they were captured.

Christians of the medieval period were assured by St. Thomas Aquinas (A.D. 1225-1274) that killing animals was sanctioned by divine providence. Perhaps Aquinas' personal habits had an effect on his opinions, for although he was a genius and an ascetic in many ways, his biographers also describe him as a glutton. Aquinas, of course, was also famous for his doctrine on the various kinds of souls a body may possess. Beasts, he taught, did not have a soul. Remarkably, according to Aquinas, neither did women. But remembering that the Church had finally relented, admitting that women do indeed have a soul,[10] Aquinas begrudgingly agreed, qualifying that they were a step above the beasts—who certainly had no soul. Many Christian leaders grew to accept this perspective.

On the other hand, if one actually studies the Bible, it becomes rather clear that animals do indeed possess a soul:

> And to every beast of the earth, and to every fowl of the air, and to everything that creepeth upon the earth, *wherein there is a living soul,* I have given every green herb for meat. (Genesis 1.30)

According to Reuben Alcalay, one of the twentieth century's greatest scholars of Hebrew-English linguistics and author of *The Complete Hebrew-English Dictionary,* the exact Hebrew words in this verse are *nefesh* ("soul") and *chayah* ("living"). Despite the fact that popular Bible translations render the above with the generic "life," and in this way try to imply that animals do not necessarily have a "soul," an accurate rendering reveals just the opposite: that animals most definitely have a soul, at least according to the Bible. What's more, the same Hebrew words are used to describe the soul of humans and even the soul of insects. Thus there is no biblical support to the argument that while animals may indeed possess some kind of soul, it is not the same kind as the one possessed by humans.

"Not By Faith Alone"

A basic tenet common to all Christians is redemption through Jesus. It is faith in being redeemed through Christ that is at the heart of Christian doctrine, not the observance of any body of specific rules and regulations, such as the law of Moses (Ephesians 2:8). It would indeed be rare to find a Christian teacher who insisted that one must or must not eat certain types of food, or that kindness to animals would affect one's salvation.

This has led to one of the major schisms in Christian theology: the faith-works polemic. While many believe that faith in Jesus is the only require-ment to attain the kingdom of God, regardless of good works or moral and ethical behavior, others feel that salvation must include faith in Jesus and good works. The idea that faith alone achieves redemption is grounded in a popular misconception of the relationship between faith and works, a misconception neatly laid bare by Rev. J. Todd Ferrier of the Order of the Cross and the English vegetarian advocate Rev. V. A. Holmes-Gore.[11]

According to both Ferrier and Holmes-Gore, the faith-works contro-versy arose when many Christian leaders of the mediaeval era began taking the teachings of Paul out of their historical context. Paul preached to the Pharisees and others who did not believe in the concept of divine grace as a redemptive force. He therefore emphasized "faith" in his teaching to the Pharisees. It is faith and works, however, that the Bible really teaches. As James says, "Faith without works is dead." (See Chapters 1 and 2 of James.) Thus, when Paul says that man can eat whatever he likes—including meat (1 Corinthians 8.8)—he is really only trying to accentuate the importance of faith.

A close study of Paul's teaching makes this clear, for despite his accen-tuation of faith, in other texts he reveals the value of righteous works, including kindness to animals. In fact, Paul taught that charitable works are even greater than faith (1 Corinthians 13:13). Still, it is all too common today to find the vast majority of the Christian community ready, willing and able to profess faith in Jesus, but not as ready to follow teachings that may require an alteration in lifestyle.

In this connection, Rev. Andrew Linzey, Chaplain of the University of Essex, has commented that many proponents of Christianity have neglected their duty to perform righteous works, especially toward the ani-mal kingdom. In his book, *Animal Rights: A Christian Assessment of Man's Treatment of Animals*, he writes with regret: "It has, I think, to be sadly rec-ognized that Christians, Catholic or otherwise, have failed to construct a satisfactory moral theology of animal treatment."[12]

However one interprets later teachings, the earliest forms of Christianity (and many of the Jewish sects from which they came) propounded the vegetarian ideal. They realized that while faith is important, proper behavior—"works"—is equally important. Thus they scrupulously followed the tenets of scripture. Not surprisingly, this affected their diet and general attitude toward animals. The Nazarenes, Therapeuts, Ebionites, Gnostics and Essenes all supported the meatless way of life. The Montanists, another early Christian sect, abstained from flesh-foods, as did Tertullian, an early Church father. Among the more orthodox fathers who disapproved of eating meat, we have already mentioned John Chrysostom and Clement of Alexandria, who were two of the most influential thinkers in the early Church.

Perhaps Clement's distinguished pupil, Origen (A.D. 185-254), one of the most prolific writers of the early Church, had the right idea about those who would endorse meat-eating: "...I believe that animal sacrifices were invented by men to be a pretext for eating flesh." (*Stromata*, *"On Sacrifices,"* *Book VII*)[13]

Later Christian sects, too, have supported vegetarianism. Ellen G. White, one of the founders of the Seventh-Day Adventist Church, was an ardent vegetarian, as was John Wesley, the founder of Methodism. Sylvester Graham, the Presbyterian minister famous for his "Graham crackers," was a propounder of the meatless ideal, and William Metcalfe, pastor of the Bible Christian Church of England, wrote a book called *Abstinence from Flesh of Animals* (1823). This is believed to be the first book on vegetarianism published in the United States.

The Trappist, Benedictine, and Carthusian Orders of the Roman Catholic Church, as well as other Christian organizations such as the Universal Christian Gnostic Movement and the Rosicrucian Fellowship, all advocate the vegetarian way of life, even if followers tend to be inconsistent in this advocacy. There are two prominent Christian groups today who work diligently to show the importance of the meatless way of life for the contemporary Christian: the Catholic Study Circle for Animal Welfare and Christians Helping Animals and People, Inc. (CHAP).

Even though Vatican II, the Ecumenical Council convened in 1965, relaxed monastic regulations in regard to meat-eating, especially for Trappist monks, most Trappists still follow the original vegetarian teachings. And although it is sometimes said that St. Francis was an inconsistent vegetarian, most Franciscan monks still practice the diet, perhaps because St. Francis is the patron saint of animals and because of his outspoken love for all of God's creatures.

A contemporary Benedictine monk, Brother David Steindl-Rast, holds that while the biblical tradition may be interpreted variously in regard to man's treatment of animals, the lives of the saints show the importance of universal compassion. Says Brother David, "Unfortunately, Christians have their share in the exploitation of our environment and in the mistreatment of animals. Sometimes they have even tried to justify their crimes by texts from the Bible, misquoted out of context. But the genuine flavor of a tradition can best be discerned in its saints....All kinds of animals appear in Christian art to distinguish one saint from another. St. Menas has two camels; St. Ulrich has a rat; St. Bridgid has ducks and geese; St. Benedict, a raven; the list goes on and on. St. Hubert's attribute is a stag with a crucifix between its antlers. According to legend, this saint was a hunter but gave up his violent ways when he suddenly saw Christ in a stag he was about to shoot."[14]

This is an eloquent example of seeing the divine in all creatures. "After all," Brother David muses, "Christ himself is called 'the lamb of God'."[15]

It is sometimes forgotten that the love endorsed by Christ is meant to be all-encompassing, a reflection of the Lord's love for all of creation. Indeed, "The Lord's Prayer" begins (in the original Aramaic): "*awoon dwashmaya.*" Although this is generally translated as "Our Father Who art in heaven," it more accurately translates into "Our *Universal* Father Who art in heaven."[16] The original Aramaic asserts that God is the Father of all living creatures in the universe, regardless of the species into which one is born. The implied meaning is that Christian love is all-embracing, and to the degree that one extends that all-embracing love, to that degree such love is returned by God. For vegetarians it is significant that "The Lord's Prayer" continues: "Give us this day our daily bread."

"Thou Shalt Not Kill"

Essential to the principle of compassion and mutual love is the Sixth Commandment: Thou shalt not kill. Although simple and direct, the commandment is rarely taken literally, and, in fact, has been traditionally interpreted as only applying to humans. Nonetheless, the exact Hebrew for Exodus 20:13, where this commandment is found, reads "lo tirtzach." According to Reuben Alcalay, the word tirtzach refers to "any kind of killing whatsoever." The exact translation, therefore, asks us to refrain from killing *in toto.*

"Thou shalt not" needs no interpretation. The controversial word is "kill," commonly defined as: 1) to deprive of life; 2) to put an end to;

3) to destroy the vital or essential quality of. If anything that has life can be killed, then an animal can be killed; according to this commandment, the killing of animals is forbidden.

Life is commonly defined as the quality that distinguishes a vital and functioning being from a dead body. Although a complex phenomenon, life manifests its presence by symptoms as recognizable to a student of the world's scriptures as to a biologist. All living entities pass through six phases: birth, growth, maintenance, reproduction, dwindling and death. An animal, then, by man's definition as well as by God's, qualifies as a living being. What is living can be killed, and to kill is to break a commandment as holy as any: "For whosoever shall keep the whole law, and yet offend in one point, he is guilty of all. For He that said, 'Do not commit adultery,' also said, 'Do not kill.' Now if thou commit no adultery, yet if thou kill, thou art become a transgressor of the law." (James 2:10,11)

There is much in the Old Testament that supports vegetarianism. It may be argued that Christians need not accept the Old Law and instead embrace only the New Testament. Jesus himself, however, taught otherwise: "Think not that I am come to destroy the law, or the prophets: I am come not to destroy, but to fulfill. For verily I say unto you, till heaven and earth pass, one jot or one tittle shall in no wise pass from the law, till all be fulfilled. Whosoever therefore shall break one of these least commandments, and shall teach men so, he shall be called the least in the kingdom of heaven. But whosoever shall do and teach them, the same shall be called great in the kingdom of God." (Matthew 5:17-19)

Interpretive Problems

Perhaps the main reason a Christian would "transgress the law," in spite of the biblical command to refrain from killing, is the widespread Christian belief that Jesus was a carnivore. Yet Jesus was known as "the Prince of Peace," and his teachings include love, compassion, and mutual respect on a universal level. It is difficult to reconcile the supremely pacifistic image of Jesus with the sanctioning of killing animals. Yet the New Testament time and again cites examples of Jesus asking for meat, which meat-eaters have taken as a sanction for their own dietary preferences. However, a close study of the original Greek reveals that Jesus did not actually ask for "meat."

Although English translations of the Gospels mention "meat" nineteen times, the original words translate more accurately into "food": *broma*— "food" (used four times); *brosimos*—"that which may be eaten" (used once);

brosis—"food, or the act of eating" (used four times); *prosphagion*—"anything to eat" (used once); *trophe*—"nourishment" (used six times); *phago*—"to eat" (used three times).

Thus, "Have ye any meat?" (John 21:5) should read: "Have ye anything to eat?" And when the Gospel says that the disciples went away to buy meat (John 4:8), a more literal translation would simply indicate that they went off to buy "food." In each case the original Greek points to "food" in general and not necessarily "meat."[17]

The problem comes down to interpretation of original material, translations and often mistranslations. Many biblical mistranslations (e.g., "Red Sea" for "Reed Sea") are inconsequential or even amusing. But some have more important ramifications, and in the cases where an incorrect version has come down through the centuries, it has become part of the biblical canon. Advocates of eating flesh can rationalize it by quotes, or misquotes, from the Bible. But if the context and tenor of the life of Jesus are taken into account, it becomes hard, if not impossible, to reconcile meat-eating with the Christian faith.

Meat-eating Christians challenge: "If the Bible encourages vegetarianism, then what about the incident of the loaves and the fishes?"

Some biblical exegetists, taking Jesus's compassionate nature into account, suggest that the "fish" were little rolls, of a kind still eaten today, made from a submarine plant known as the fish plant, which grows in the East. These soft fish plants are dried in the sun, ground into flour in a mortar, and baked into rolls. Fish-plant rolls were an integral part of the ancient Babylonian diet, and many Japanese, too, consider them a great delight. The Muslims recommend that the faithful eat them and, most important, they were a popular delicacy in Jesus's time. Then, too, there is a practical matter to be considered: in a basket also containing bread, there would more likely be rolls than fish, which would spoil rapidly in hot weather and ruin any other food in the basket.[18]

It is also possible that "bread and fish" had a symbolic rather than literal sense, not unusual in sacred writings. Bread is a symbol of Christ's body, or the Divine Substance, and "fish" was a password in the early Church, when the Christians had to conceal their identity to avoid persecution. The letters of the Greek word for fish, I-CH-TH-U-S, are also the initial letters of *Iesous Christos Theou Uios Soter* ("Jesus Christ, Son of God, Savior").[19] Thus, the fish assumed a mystical symbolism in Christianity, and its use can be seen on the walls of the Roman catacombs.

Most importantly, there is no reference to fish in the earliest New Testament manuscripts; the miracle is described as bread and fruit, not loaves and fish. It was the later Bible manuscripts (after the fourth century) that list fish instead of fruit. The Codex Sinaiticus is the earliest edition of the New Testament to mention fish as a part of that miracle.

Still, there are those who cannot dispense with the traditional example of the loaves and the fishes. For such people, it should be noted that even if Jesus did eat fish, he offered no sanction for others to do so in his name. Jesus lived among and preached to fishermen. As a teacher, he had to consider his audience and circumstances. Thus, he told his disciples to throw down their fishing nets and instead to become "fishers of men," or preachers. Still, those who speak of Jesus's eating fish say, "Jesus did this, so why can't I?" But when we consider how Jesus gave his very life to preach the glories of God, few are enthusiastic to follow his example.

The Paschal Lamb

While there is familiar symbolism in Jesus as the Good Shepherd and as the lamb of God, the Paschal Lamb offers a problem for vegetarian Christians. Was the Last Supper a Passover meal in which Jesus and the Apostles feasted on the flesh of a lamb?

The Synoptic (first three) Gospels say that the Last Supper was the Passover meal, which would imply that Jesus and his followers ate the Passover lamb (Matthew 26:17, Mark 16:16, Luke 22:13). John, however, says that the Last Supper took place earlier: "Now before the feast of Passover, Jesus knowing that his hour was come...riseth from supper and layeth aside his garments; and he took a towel and girded himself." (John 13:1-4) But if the time sequence were different, then the Last Supper would not have been a Passover meal.

In his excellent book, *Why Kill for Food?*, English historian Geoffrey Rudd analyzes the problem of the Paschal Lamb in the following way. The Last Supper took place on a Thursday evening; the Crucifixion, on the very next day, Friday. However, according to the Jewish perspective, these two events occur on the same day, as the Jewish full day begins at sundown of the previous evening. Naturally, this gets quite confusing. In Chapter 19 of his Gospel, John says that the Crucifixion took place on the day of the preparation of the Passover, which would be Thursday. Later, in verse 31, he says that the body of Jesus was not left on the cross because "the day of that Sabbath was a high day." In other words, the Passover, on the Sabbath, began at sundown that Friday, after the Crucifixion.

Although the first three Gospels contradict John's version, which most biblical scholars consider an accurate account, in other passages they support it. In Matthew 26:5, for instance, the priests say that they will not kill Jesus during the feast "lest a tumult arise among the people." On the other hand, the Gospel of Matthew elsewhere puts the Last Supper and the Crucifixion on the day of the Passover. Furthermore, it must be noted that according to Talmudic custom there would be no question of holding trials and executing people on the first and holiest days of Passover.

The Passover being as holy as the Sabbath, the Jews would not carry weapons if it had begun (Mark 14:43, 47), nor would they buy linen and spices for the burial (Mark 15:46, Luke 23:56). Finally, the haste with which the disciples put Jesus in the tomb is consistent with their desire that his body be removed from the cross before the Passover began (Mark 15:42-46).

Actually, the lamb is conspicuous by its absence: it is never even mentioned in connection with the Last Supper. The biblical historian J. A. Gleizes suggests that in substituting bread and wine for flesh and blood in the divine sacrifice Jesus announced the new alliance between man and God, "a true reconciliation with all His creatures."[20] If Jesus had been a meat-eater, he would have used a lamb and not bread as the symbol of the Divine Passion, in which the Lamb of God is slain for the sins of the world. All evidence indicates that the Last Supper was not the Passover supper with its traditional lamb, but rather it was a "farewell meal" that Jesus lovingly shared with his disciples. This was confirmed by the late Rev. Charles Gore, Bishop of Oxford: "We will assume John is right when he corrects Mark as to the nature of the Last Supper. It was not the Paschal Meal proper, but a supper observed as a farewell supper with His disciples. Nor do the accounts of the supper suggest the ceremonial of the Passover meal." (*A New Commentary on Holy Scripture*, part three, p. 235)[21]

Conclusion

Based on literal translations of the earliest Christian texts, there is no instance where meat-eating is condoned or accepted. Much of the later Christian rationalization for the eating of flesh is based on mistranslations or a literal interpretation of common Christian symbolism that was meant in a figurative sense. The key element is, of course, interpretation, and one must weigh the actions of Jesus and his disciples to see if they are at all reconcilable with a meat-centered diet. Further, the early Christian fathers and sects practiced strict vegetarianism. Thus, by careful biblical translation, extrapolation of the broader context of Jesus's teachings, and the explicit teachings of the early Christians, we see the espousal of vegetarianism.

This ideal of living in harmony with all of God's creatures was beautifully expressed in a poem by Werner Bergengruen, which tells of a dog who strays into a church during Mass. Upset and nervous, the little girl to whom the dog belongs manages to pull her canine friend out of the church. "What an embarrassment," she thinks, "an animal in the church!" But Bergengruen points out that the church is full of animals: ox and ass at the Christmas crib, a lion at the feet of St. Jerome, Jonah's fish, St. Martin's mount, the eagle, the dove, and even the serpent. From pictures and statues all over the church, animals start smiling as the little girl bashfully realizes that her pet is one among many. The organist laughs and then sings: "Praise God all, all ye creatures!" Such praise is natural, for in the church, as everywhere else, all beings come from God.

Thus, the great Franciscan order, for instance, celebrated the unity of creation by stressing the fact of common origin. "When he [St. Francis] considered the primordial source of all things," wrote St. Bonaventure, "he was filled with even more abundant piety, calling creatures no matter how small, by the name of brother or sister, because he knew they had the same source as himself."[22] This is the perfection of Christian love.

REFERENCES

1. The reference here, which describes the animal exacting revenge upon its human predator, coincides precisely with the law of action and reaction (karma) and is completely consistent with the Sanskrit word *mamsa* ("meat"), which is described in the section on Hinduism.
2. Gnostic Orthodox Church, *The Four Soul Killers* (Oklahoma, St. George Press, 1979), p.15.
3. Joseph Benson, *The Holy Bible, Containing the Old and New Testaments* (New York, T. Mason & G. Lane Pub., 1839), Vol. 1, p. 43.
4. Etienne de Courcelles, *Diatriba de esu sanguinis inter Christianos* ("Discourse Concerning the Eating of Blood Among Christians"); see *Opera theologica* ("Theological Works"), Amsterdam, 1675, p. 971.
5. Eusebius, *The Ecclesiastical History*, V. i. 26, Loeb Classical Library (Cambridge and London, Harvard University Press, 1980), p. 419.
6. Charles Joseph Hefele, *A History of the Councils of the Church, From the Original Documents* (Edinburgh, T. & T. Clark Pub., 1896), p. 232.
7. St. John Chrysostom, Homily 69 (On Matthew 22:1-4), trans. George Prevost, *Nicene and Post-Nicene Fathers*, series 1, ed. P. Schaft, W. B. Eerdmans (Grand Rapids, Mich.), Vol. 10, 1956, p. 425.
8. Titus Flavius Clemens, *Paidagogos* (The Instructor), Book 2, *Ante-Nicene Fathers*, ed. A. Roberts and J. Donaldson, W. B. Eerdmans (Grand Rapids, Mich.), Vol. 2, 1967, p. 241.
9. Upton C. Ewing, *The Essene Christ* (New York, Philosophical Library, 1961), p. 85.
10. The Synod of Macon (A.D. 585) was convened largely to decide whether or not women have souls. Perhaps the Church would do well to hold a council in regard to animals.
11. See Rev. V. A. Holmes-Gore, *These We Have Not Loved* (London, The C. W. Daniel Company, Ltd., 1946), pp. 99-100.
12. Andrew Liney, *Animal Rights: A Christian Assessment of Man's Treatment of Animals* (London, SCM Press, 1976), pp. 4-5.
13. Quoted in J. Todd Ferrier, *On Behalf of the Creatures* (London, The Order of the Cross, 1968), p. 19.
14. An Interview with Brother David Steindl-Rast, "A Christian View of Animals," *Buddhists Concerned for Animals* newsletter, San Francisco, Vol. 5, p. 9.
15. *Ibid.*
16. Rocco A. Errico, *The Ancient Aramaic Prayer of Jesus* (Los Angeles, Science of Mind Pub., 1978), p. 24.
17. G. L. Rudd, *Why Kill for Food?* (Madras, Indian Vegetarian Congress, 1956), p. 87.
18. *Ibid.* p. 92.
19. *Ibid.*
20. *Ibid.* pp. 89-90.
21. *Ibid.*
22. St. Bonaventure in *The Classics of Western Spirituality: Bonaventure—The Life of St. Francis*, trans. Ewert Cousins (New York, Paulist Press, 1978), pp. 254-5.

EARLY CHRISTIANITY

Chapter 2

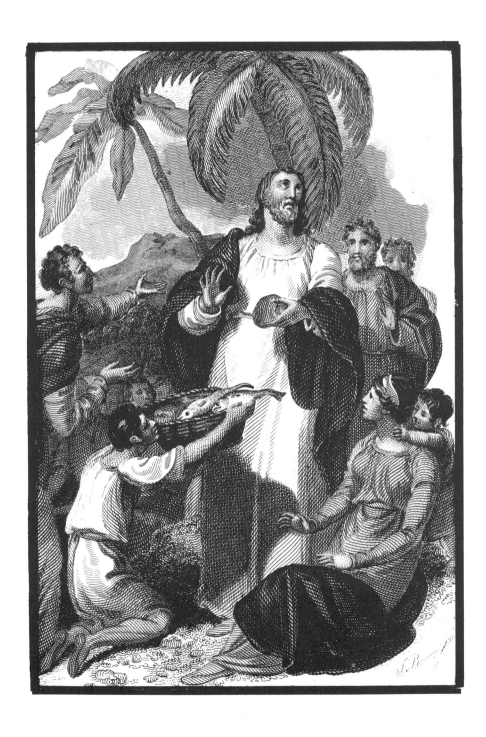

EARLY CHRISTIANITY

"And the flesh of slain beasts in his body
will become his own tomb.
For I tell you truly, he who kills, kills himself,
and whoso eats the flesh of slain beasts,
eats the body of death."

—The Essene Gospel of Peace

The previous chapter dealt with vegetarianism and the traditional Christian heritage with which most people are accustomed. This chapter will be devoted to what today may seem a form of "radical" Christianity, based on the Dead Sea Scrolls and other relatively recent findings of the Christian Era. (These findings, it should be noted, are not actually "radical," but rather the embodiment of the earliest forms of Christianity, closest to what Jesus preached.) This book neither promotes nor rejects the Dead Sea Scrolls, Nag Hammadi or other documents in question. As in the previous chapter, our purpose will be to see what light these early scrolls shed on vegetarianism in the Christian tradition. While the preceding chapter dealt largely with the premise that the Bible has not been changed, this chapter assumes that it has.

Many scholars assert that at the Council of Nicea (A.D. 325) priests and politicians completely altered original Christian documents, through omission and interpolation, in order to make them acceptable to Emperor Constantine, who, at the time, bitterly opposed the scriptures.[1] Their purpose was to convert Constantine to Christianity and thus make their religion the accepted creed of the Roman Empire.

"Some are not aware," wrote Archdeacon Wilderforce, "that, after the Council of Nicea, the manuscripts of the New Testament were considerably tampered with. Professor Nestle, in his Introduction to the Textual Criticism of the Greek Testament, tells us that certain scholars, called 'correctores,' were appointed by the ecclesiastical authorities, and were actually commissioned to correct the text of the scripture in the interest of what was considered orthodox."[2]

Commenting on this idea in the Foreword to his translation of *The Gospel of the Holy Twelve,* Rev. Gideon Jasper Richard Ousley says: "What these correctores did was to cut out of the Gospels, with minute care, certain teachings of our Lord which they did not propose to follow—namely, those against the eating of flesh and the taking of strong drink..."[3]

Early Texts

The Dead Sea Scrolls—biblical manuscripts that date back to the beginning of the Christian Era—were discovered in 1947 and tend to support the view that the Bible has been changed, especially in regard to practices such as meat-eating. The value of these scrolls (and that of other archaeological finds since that year) lies in the possibility of their being original, unchanged manuscripts that date back to the time of Jesus. The only other New Testament documents available date from the fourth century (at the earliest), and these are only copies of copies. Although some scholars claim that there are no glaring differences between the Dead Sea findings and later Bible documents, it is undeniable that many of these texts are marked by subtle but meaningful differences.

While some Christian historians reject these archaeological finds, others put great faith in them. Among these, Dr. Martin Larson, Edmond B. Szekely, Millar Burrows, G. J. Ousley, John M. Allegro and Frank J. Muccie (founder of the Edenite Society) have made substantial contributions in uncovering early Christian texts, and from these works we have come to know about vegetarianism in the early Christian tradition.

Ousley, for example, has composed a translation of what purports to be the original Gospels, preserved by members of the Essene community (a religious sect whose members lived in the Dead Sea area and are remembered for their discipline and spiritual integrity). Ousley relates that the manuscript had been preserved in a Tibetan Buddhist monastery, "where it was hidden by some of the Essene community for safety from the hands of the corrupters..."[4]

If authentic, Ousley's manuscripts would be the most ancient and complete Christian writings in existence: an original Aramaic text unchanged since its use in the first Christian church of Jerusalem. Those scholars who accept the text as authentic conclude that it was the original Gospel on which the four Gospels of the New Testament are based (with numerous variations and important omissions). This may or may not be true, but the information delineated in these manuscripts is clearly supportive of the vegetarian ideal, and thus worthy of scrutiny here.

It is interesting that just before his death, Ousley expressed concern over the future of the manuscript: what had happened in the past might happen again. In all probability, Ousley thought, it would happen, especially if the manuscript were put under the editorship of materialists, in whose hands "correction" would become "corruption." As a precaution, in 1904 Ousley transferred the copyright to his work to a trusted friend with the request "not to let it get into the hands of ritualists, whether Roman or Anglican."[5] Ousley's treasured manuscript, called *The Gospel of the Holy Twelve*, previously known as *The Gospel to the Hebrews* and sometimes *The Nazarene Gospel*, survives to this day.[6]

Excerpts on Kindness to Animals

According to *The Gospel of the Holy Twelve*, before Jesus's birth, the angel told Mary: "Ye shall eat no flesh nor take strong drink, for the child shall be consecrated unto God from his mother's womb, and neither flesh nor strong drink shall he take." The strength of such a heavenly command, if it is accepted as historical record, would be in its confirmation of Jesus as the messiah of Old Testament prophecy: "Therefore the Lord Himself shall give you a sign. Behold, a young woman shall conceive, and bear a son, and his name shall be called Emmanuel. He shall eat butter and honey, that he may know to refuse evil, and to choose the good." (Isaiah 7:14, 15)

The text continues to describe that the community in which Joseph and Mary lived did not slaughter a lamb in celebrating the feast of the Passover: "Now Joseph and Mary, his parents, went up to Jerusalem every year at the feast of the Passover, and observed the feast after the manner of their brethren, who abstained from bloodshed and the eating of flesh..."

This description of his community would help explain why, from childhood, Jesus loved birds and animals: "And on a certain day the child Jesus came to a place where a snare was set for birds and there were some boys there. And Jesus said to them, 'Who hath set this snare for these innocent creatures of God? Behold, in a snare will they in like manner be caught.'"

In these reputedly untampered texts, it is not surprising that Jesus teaches us to be considerate of all creatures and not of man alone: "Be ye therefore considerate, be tender, be pitiful, be kind, not to your kind alone, but to every creature which is within your care; for ye are to them as gods, to whom they look in their needs."

Jesus goes on to explain that he has come to end the blood sacrifices: "I am come to end the sacrifices and feasts of blood; and if ye cease not offering and eating of flesh and blood, the wrath of God shall not cease from you; even as it came to your fathers in the wilderness, who lusted for flesh, and did eat to their content, and were filled with rottenness, and the plague consumed them."

The miracle of the loaves and fishes, as mentioned in the preceding chapter, is not found in these early manuscripts. Instead, there is a description of a miracle of bread, fruit, and a pitcher of water. "And Jesus set the bread and the fruit before them, and also the water. And they did eat and drink—and were filled. And they marveled; for each had enough and to spare, and there were four thousand. And they departed, thanking God for what they had heard and seen."

These early documents have Jesus endorsing a natural diet time and again, especially vegetarianism: "And on hearing these things, a certain Sadducee, who believed not in the holy things of God, asked Jesus, 'Tell me, please, why sayest thou, do not eat the flesh of animals. Were not the beasts given unto man as food, even as the fruits and herbs ye spoke of?' Jesus answered him and said, 'Behold this melon, the fruit of the earth.' And Jesus broke open a watermelon and further said unto the Sadducee, 'See thou with thine own eyes the good fruit of the soil, the meat of man, and see thou the seeds within, count ye them, for one melon maketh a hundredfold and even more. If thou sow this seed, ye do eat from the true God, for no blood was spilled, nay, no pain nor outcry did ye hear with thy ears or see with thine eyes. The true food of man is from the mother of the earth, for she brings forth perfect gifts unto the humble of the land. But ye seek what Satan giveth, the anguish, the death, and the blood of living souls taken by the sword. Know ye not, those who live by the sword are the ones who die by the same death? Go ye thine way then, and plant the seeds of the good fruit of life, and leave ye off from hurting the innocent creatures of God.'"

Jesus even condemns those who hunt animals: "And as Jesus was walking along with some of his disciples, they met up with a certain man who trained dogs to hunt other weaker creatures. And seeing this, Jesus said to the man, 'Why doest thou this foul thing?' And the man answered and said, 'By this I earn my living; for what purpose do these creatures profit anything? Yea, these creatures are weak, and deserve death, but the dogs, they are strong.'

"And Jesus looked upon the man with a sad countenance and said, 'Thou truly lacketh wisdom and love from above, for lo, every creature which God hath made, hath its own end and purpose in the kingdom of life, and who can say what good is there in it? Or what profit to thyself, or mankind? For it is not thy part to judge the weak as inferior to the strong, for the weak were not delivered unto man as food or for sport....Woe to the crafty who hurt and destroy the creatures of God! Yea, woe to the hunters, for they will be hunted, and with what mercy they shew unto their innocent prey, the same will they receive at the hands of unworthy men! Leave off from this foul work of evil men, work what is good in the eyes of the Lord and be blessed, lest ye be cursed on thy own account.'"

Finally, in these early manuscripts we read that Jesus actually rebukes the fishermen, despite the fact that they were his strongest supporters: "And on another day, the question of eating dead things was again presented, and some of Jesus's newer disciples gathered around him and asked, 'Master, ye do indeed know all things, and thy wisdom of the Holy Law excels all others; tell us, therefore, is the eating of sea creatures lawful as some say?'

"And Jesus looked upon them with sad eyes, for he knew they were yet unlearned men and their hearts were yet hardened by false doctrines of devils; and he said unto them: 'See ye the fish of the sea, as we stand beside the seashore and look upon the waters of many lives. Yea, the water is their world, even as the dry land belongeth to man; I ask thee, do the fish come unto thee and ask of thee for thy dry land or of its foods? Nay. Nor is it lawful for thee to go into the sea and ask for things which belong not unto thee; for the earth is divided into three kingdoms of souls—one of the land, one of the air, and one of the sea, each according to its kind. And deposition for the Eternal Being hath given unto them each the spirit of life and the Holy Breath, and what He giveth freely unto His creatures, neither men nor angels have authority to take back or claim as their own.'"

Interestingly, when Jesus first instructs his disciples, who were Jews, about their newly adopted diet (vegetarianism), they criticize him: "Thou speakest against the Law"—evidently referring to permission in various parts of the Old Testament that allowed them to eat meat. Jesus's memorable response to this is quite revealing: "Against Moses indeed I do not speak, nor against the Law, which he permitted for the hardness of your hearts. Verily, I say unto you, in the beginning all creatures of God did find their sustenance in the herbs and the fruits of the earth alone, until the ignorance and selfishness of man turned many of them to that which was contrary to their original use; but even these shall yet return to their natural food; as it is written in the prophets, and their words shall not fail."

These excerpts, among others, can be found in *The Humane Gospel of Jesus*, published by the Edenite Society. It is one of the few English translations of *The Gospel of the Holy Twelve*. Whether one accepts with faith the teachings of these Essene texts or dismisses them as disreputable forgeries, the teachings themselves appear wholly consonant with the fundamental teachings of Jesus Christ, for they are based on the ultimate achievement in love and compassion.

REFERENCES

1. *The Edenite Creed for Life* (N.J., The Edenite Society, 1979), p. 19.
2. *Ibid.*
3. *The Gospel of the Holy Twelve* (CA, Health Research, Reprint: 1974), p. 8.
4. *Ibid.*
5. *Ibid.*
6. *The Essene Humane Gospel of Jesus* (N.J., The Edenite Society, 1978), p. 6.

JUDAISM
Chapter 3

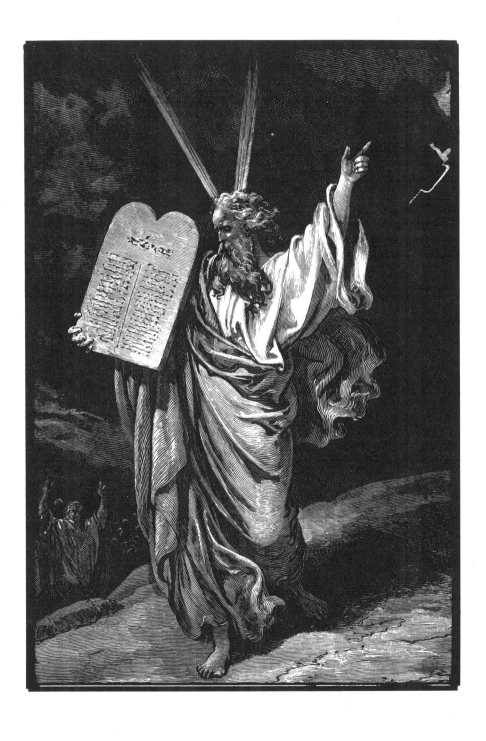

JUDAISM

"You who have compassion for a lamb
shall be the shepherd of my people Israel."
—Exodus Rabbah 2, Midrash

Today, orthodox Judaism does not generally teach that vegetarianism is a scriptural principle. Of course, the scriptures do inform us that each generation of Jews has a lesser understanding of Torah than its predecessor (*Tractate Berakhot*, 20A, *Talmud Bavli*). This may account for modern Judaism's denial of the vegetarian way of life. After all, the first diet given to man in the Torah (also known as the Old Testament or the Five Books of Moses) is clearly vegetarian:

> I have given you every herb-bearing seed, which is upon the face of all the earth and every tree, in which is the fruit of a tree-yielding seed: to you it shall be for food... (Genesis 1:29)

Genesis 3:18 added the further instruction to eat vegetables. In obedience to these injunctions, the people of Israel—for ten generations (from Adam to Noah)—were frugivorous and vegetarian.

However, this adherence to God's law was short-lived. By the time of Noah, morality had diminished considerably. Animal sacrifice began (Genesis 4:4), animal skins were now used as clothing (Genesis 3:21), and human beings began to murder one another (Genesis 4:8, 23). It was during this period of "falling into sin," as the Bible describes it, that God gave concessions for the eating of flesh-foods. Meat-eating became rampant.

43

After the great flood had destroyed all vegetation, God issued a tempo-rary sanction to eat meat (Genesis 9:4). Shortly thereafter, however, God again attempted to institute a vegetarian diet. When the Israelites left Egypt, God provided *manna*, a non-flesh food meant to sustain them dur-ing their arduous journey. Still, the Israelites demanded meat, and God supplied it—along with a fatal plague for all who ate it (this is described in Numbers 11:18-34 and in this book's chapter on Christianity). Meat-eating had by now become thoroughly ingrained and widespread among the Jewish people, and the Bible indicates that God, after two attempts at instituting vegetarianism, was ready to permit meat-eating, with certain restrictions.

Dominion

Mankind was given "dominion" over all of creation (Genesis 1:26), and many adherents of the Judaeo-Christian tradition refer to this dominion in an attempt to rationalize the killing and eating of animals. Dr. Richard Schwartz insightfully lays all such attempts to rest in his *Judaism and Vegetarianism:*

> Dominion does not mean that we have the right to conquer and exploit. Immediately after God gave people dominion over animals (Genesis 1:26), he prohibited their use for food (Genesis 1:29). Dominion means guardianship or stewardship—being co-workers with God in taking care of and improving the world.
> The Talmud interprets "dominion" as the privilege of using animals for labor only. It is extremely doubtful that the concept of dominion permits breeding animals and treating them as machines designed solely to meet our needs.
> Rabbi Kook states that dominion does not in any way imply the rule of a haughty despot who tyrannically governs for his own personal selfish ends and with a stubborn heart. He states that he cannot believe that such a repulsive form of servitude could be forever sealed in the world of God, Whose "tender mercies are over all His works."
> Rabbi Hirsch stresses that people have not been given the right or the power to have all subservient to them. In commenting on Genesis 1:26 he states, "The earth and its creatures may have other relationships of which we are ignorant, in which they serve their own purpose." Thus, above people's control over nature, there is a Divine control to serve God's purposes and objectives, and people have no right to interfere. Hence, people, according to Judaism, do not have an unlimited right to use and abuse animals and other parts of nature.[1]

This is further confirmed in the mediaeval work *Sefer Chasidim* ("The Book of the Pious"), which states, "Be kind and compassionate to all creatures that the Holy One, blessed be He, created in this world. Never beat nor inflict pain on any animal, beast, bird or insect. Do not throw stones at a dog or a cat, nor should ye kill flies or wasps." Accordingly, many Jewish heroes and heroines were singled out by God because of their compassion for animals. In the Midrash, for instance, it is said that Moses was deemed worthy to lead the Jews out of Egypt because he showed compassion to a lamb. And it is pointed out that Rebekah was selected for Isaac's wife because she exhibited kindness to thirsty camels.

Still, as Judaism expanded and grew, so did the desire for the flesh of animals. To this end, convenient interpretations of "man's dominion" became popular and other scriptural concepts to endorse meat-eating were invented.

The Dietary Laws

In an attempt to accommodate the growing demand for the flesh of animals, dietary laws were soon decreed. Rabbi Abraham Isaac Kook (1865-1935), the first Chief Rabbi of Modern Israel, articulated the feelings of many Jewish thinkers when he conjectured that these restrictions over eating meat were imposed by God to minimize the slaughter of animals. Much earlier, the great Jewish philosopher Moses Maimonides (1135-1204) had stated that animal sacrifice was a substitute for child sacrifice, a widespread practice among ancient peoples. Still, all meat was to be offered at the Temple, which was destroyed in A.D. 70. Today, there are complex laws for koshering meats and making them acceptable for a Jewish household.

It is interesting that the Jewish dietary laws apply only to animal foods. All fruits, vegetables, unprocessed grains and cereals, and even dairy products are kosher. Only meat must be prepared in a special way. Further, according to Rabbi Samuel H. Dresner, in his classic work, *The Jewish Dietary Laws*,

> Kashrut [the dietary law] teaches, first of all, that the eating of meat is itself a sort of compromise....Man ideally should not eat meat, for to eat meat a life must be taken, an animal must be put to death....The Torah [thus] teaches a lesson in moral conduct, that man shall not eat meat unless he has a special craving for it, and shall eat it only occasionally and sparingly (Chulin 84a)... [2]

The Rabbi goes on to explain that meat-eating is a "divine concession," an extreme measure to deal with human selfishness and ineptitude. But God makes clear the importance of revering all life, the Rabbi tells us, citing many examples from scripture: "Animals are allowed to rest on the Sabbath." (Exodus 23:12) "Ploughing with a bull and a donkey harnessed together was forbidden because they were not equal in strength and the weaker would suffer in trying to keep up with the stronger." (Deut. 22:10) "If a man finds a nest of birds, he cannot take the mother bird and the young: he first has to send away the mother to spare her feelings." (Deut. 22:6) "While treading out the corn, the ox (or any other animal) cannot be muzzled." (Deut. 25:4) According to Jewish tradition, Rabbi Dresner concludes, "When an animal is born, it is not to be taken away from its mother for at least seven days."[3] Using these exhortations to mercy as examples, Dresner points out that the Bible teaches reverence for all life.

This state in which one feels regard for all creatures has been described by Jewish scholars as the "Edenic" state, for it was embraced by the first people in the Garden of Eden. There is a Jewish tradition, furthermore, which holds that man will again reach that Edenic state when the messiah comes. Accordingly, to approach a new and higher level of spiritual grandeur, many Jewish thinkers have already adopted vegetarianism in preparation for the messiah's appearance.[4]

For instance, Shlomo Goren, the former Chief Ashkenazi Rabbi of Israel, is a devout vegetarian. Reputed as one of the greatest existential philosophers and modern Jewish thinkers, Martin Buber (1878-1965) also advocated a meatless diet. Isaac Bashevis Singer, who won the 1978 Nobel Prize for Literature, and Shmuel Yoseph Agnon, another Nobel Prize winner, are both Jewish authors who support the doctrine of kindness to animals as underlying the basis of their vegetarianism. Rabbi David Rosen, the former Chief Rabbi of Ireland, and Shear Yashuv Cohen, the Chief Rabbi of Haifa, are tremendously supportive of the vegetarian way of life. The late Chief Rabbi Kook, although inconsistent in his own practice, actively spoke out in favor of vegetarianism. His Hebrew booklet, *The Vision of Vegetarianism and Peace,* is one of the most convincing and thought-provoking pieces on Jewish vegetarianism.

The list of prominent Jewish vegetarians—both secular and religious—goes on, and one need hardly doubt that vegetarianism fits securely into the Jewish way of life; that it is, in fact, preferable. Nonetheless, dietary laws exist for those who may desire to eat meat, although indiscriminate meat-eating is never approved in the Jewish tradition.

In Jewish dietary law, certain animals are designated "clean," or fit for human consumption, whereas others are "unclean," meaning that they should not be eaten. The listing of clean and unclean animals can be found in Chapter 11 of Leviticus and Chapter 14 of Deuteronomy. There it states that all fruits and vegetables are for the use of man. The animals permitted for consumption must be herbivorous—that is to say, plant-eaters, not meat-eaters—and they must have cloven hooves and chew cud. All predators, animals or birds, were proscribed as not fit for human consumption. Also counted as unclean, incidentally, is the carcass of any clean animal not ritually slaughtered. One of the more curious laws is that any person who merely touches such a carcass is made "unclean" until evening.

Historically, Jews who strictly followed ritualistic prescriptions refused, as a matter of religious principle, to search for the objective reasons why certain animals could be eaten and others could not. This is the attitude of many contemporary orthodox Jews as well. For them, the Jewish way of life has been set down by the forefathers—and this is all that one need know. The details require no probing. Others—Jews trained in philosophy, scholars of comparative religion (especially those of the Greco-Roman Era and the Middle Ages)—felt the need to reconcile their faith with the dictates of reason. As the Psalms (47:7) inform us: "Sing ye praises with understanding." Let us then pursue proper understanding.

In the third century before the Common Era, we find the Jewish scholar Aristeas critically examining the dietary laws which, he stated, had been given to the Jews to inculcate in them the spirit of justice and to awaken pious reflections. To prove his contention, he pointed to the fact that in kashrut (Jewish dietary laws), birds of prey are forbidden as food so the Jew might recall the first principle of social justice: not to prey on others.

About two centuries later, Philo of Alexandria, who was a Platonist philosopher as well as a rabbi, attempted to interpret scriptural law by the method of allegory, assigning a human vice to every creature branded in the Bible as "unclean," and reading into every prohibition a devout exhortation to humans to take themselves in hand and master their "unclean" passions and habits.

Rav Yoseph Albo (c. A.D. 1500), the great Jewish mystic, in his work *Sefer Ha'Ikkarim*, boldly claims that it was God's acknowledgment of sheer human weakness that led Him to permit humans to eat meat. Albo refers to the Cain and Abel story and argues that when Cain saw Abel kill an animal for a sacrifice—and receive a reward—Cain assumed that killing was permissible. Cain, Albo states, "conveniently interpreted" the whole affair. Albo warns us not to do the same.

According to Rabbi James M. Lebeau, co-chairman of the United Synagogue of America's Central Youth Commission, "Both Maimonides and Nahmanides (A.D. 1194-1270) praised vegetarianism, yet they concluded that human beings could eat meat as long as they introduced humane slaughtering procedures."[5]

Author Richard Schwartz calls for Jews to see beyond a mere "humane" form of slaughter. Says Schwartz:

> Certainly *shechita* [Jewish technique of animal slaughter] provides for the most humane slaughter. But can conscientious Jews consider only the final seconds of an animal's life and ignore months and perhaps years of terribly cruel conditions? Can a religion which mandates that the ox and ass should not be yoked together (Deut. 22:10), that the ox should not be muzzled while threshing in the fields (Deut. 25:4), and that animals are to be free to graze in open fields and enjoy the beauties of creation on the sabbath (Rashi, commentary on Exodus 23:12), ignore widespread violations of *tsa-ar ba-ale chayim*, the command to avoid inflicting pain on living creatures?[6]

Schwartz's point is well taken, especially in light of today's factory farming techniques, which torture the animals long before their death. But even with the ostensibly humane techniques of kosher slaughter, animals are still forced to endure suffering. The English Royal Society for the Prevention of Cruelty to Animals (RSPCA) has this to say:

> ...the Jewish and Moslem communities are exempt from the law that requires all animals to be stunned before they are slaughtered....Since neither Jews nor Moslems eat pork, religious slaughter is confined to cattle, sheep, goats and poultry. In the case of cattle...the animal is placed in a restraining device called a 'Weinberg Pen.' This is a metal crate, in which the cow or steer is held, and which is slowly revolved until the animal is upside down. The cow's or steer's neck is then extended and the throat cut. Sheep and goats are picked up and placed on their backs in a metal cradle before their throats are cut. Poultry are held head downwords, usually restrained only by hand, before cutting the throat.[7]

With just as much compassion as accuracy, the RSPCA concludes,

> There is very often a time-lag of anything from seventeen seconds to six minutes from the moment the animal's throat is cut until it actually loses consciousness. Obviously, this is a very long time indeed to an animal in pain and terror. The reason for this lengthy duration between the throat being cut and consciousness being lost may be due either to the continuing

blood supply to the brain through the unsevered vertebral artery, and/or failure to cut both carotid arteries which supply blood to the head. Thus, although the throat may be cut, the animal is by no means free from pain and can in some cases have a considerable awareness of what is happening to it.[8]

There is no such thing as "humane" slaughter. And to eat animals, one has to slaughter them.

However, Rabbi Shneur Zalman of Liady (1748-1812), the mystic who founded the Lubavitch sect, had his own view of meat-eating, unfortunately trying to elevate it to a divine principle. He taught that all the world exists for the greater glory of God. If a God-fearing individual, the Rabbi taught, eats meat or drinks wine in order to have strength to serve God—then the flesh that he eats goes up to the Almighty as a sacrifice. In other words, if a cow, for example, lives and dies a normal life, then it was just a cow. But if it is slaughtered and then eaten by a "religious person," then the cow becomes something higher than itself. In giving its life to become food for such a person, the cow becomes elevated to a level of divine service. From this perspective, killing and eating animals is not to their detriment, but rather it raises them to a sort of advanced life form, a sacrificial being. While there is certainly a logic to this, it is up to each individual Jew to decide whether God wants an animal sacrifice, or one that does not involve killing.

Perhaps the Bible will help determine one's decision: "I will have mercy, and not sacrifice." (Hosea 6:6) Or further, "When you make many prayers, I will hear not: your hands are full of blood." (Isaiah 1:15)

Kosher Meats

The Fourth Commandment, ordaining the seventh day (Sabbath) as the day of rest for the Jews, includes beasts as well as people. The Babylonian Talmud even established the rule that before a man could sit down to his meal, he first was obligated to feed his animals—because they could not help themselves. Further, the Talmud states that to save an animal's life, or even to relieve it of pain, one is allowed to break any ordinance of Sabbath observance (and it should be noted that the Jews consider the Sabbath their holiest day). In fact, Jewish tradition reveals that the extensive regulations that order ritual slaughtering of animals, the *shechitah* and kosher laws, were originally motivated by simple humane considerations: to cause the animal as little pain as possible. Vegetarianism is, therefore, the logical extension of Jewish dietary law, which exists to spare animals pain. Obviously, one would cause the least amount of pain possible (to animals) by giving up meat-eating altogether.

For those who would not give up meat, however, koshering laws were enacted. Central to these laws is a process that drains the blood from the animals. The reason for this is the biblical commandment that we abstain from eating the blood of animals and fowl. This commandment is repeated several times in the Old Testament (e.g., Genesis 9:4; Leviticus 17:14; Deuteronomy 12:16). Talmudic literature goes so far as to say that the soul or life-force is to be found in the blood. This is also a concept found in early Hinduism, which avers that as the heart pumps the blood throughout the body, it also pumps the symptom of the life-force—consciousness. Thus, the blood is considered sacred.

To remove the blood from the meat effectively, early rabbinical authorities devised a means by which the meat is first soaked in water to open the pores and then salted to draw out the blood. When this is done under rabbinical supervision—with the animal first having been slaughtered according to the *shechitah,* or "humane" procedure—an observant Jew will then consume meat products with the firm belief that it is now "kosher," or acceptable to God. The process is defective, however, in that the long and rigorous koshering system never actually achieves its end: all the blood is never drained out. It would be more consistent with the Jewish tradition, then, to adhere to a vegetarian diet, for the vegetarian does not eat any blood.

Vegetarianism has also filtered down to contemporary Jewish texts, as in this passage from the *Haggadah for the Liberated Lamb* : "...vegetarianism is less a break with tradition than a return to an historical trend."[9] The Haggadah concludes: "...there is no commandment to eat meat in the Bible, nor is there any blessing to be said for the eating of animal flesh."[10] *The Encyclopedia Judaica* adds, "...meat is never included among the staple diet of the children of Israel, which is confined to agricultural products, of which the constantly recurring expression in the Bible is 'grain and wine and oil' (Deut. 11:14) or the seven agricultural products enumerated in Deuteronomy 8:8."[11] Even though meat was not considered a staple, it gradually became a favorite among religious Jews who could afford it. Kashrut, the koshering laws, gave meat-eating a divine basis.

A simplified form of the koshering process is listed here:

> 1. Before the meat is salted, it must be thoroughly washed in water. The meat must be entirely submerged in water for half an hour. If the water

is very cold, it should be put in a warm place before the meat is soaked in it, because meat becomes hardened in cold water and the blood will not easily emerge.

2. After the meat is washed thoroughly, it should soak in water for a short time. When the water no longer becomes reddened by the blood, the meat should be salted.

3. Frozen meat must be allowed to thaw out before being soaked, yet it must not be placed near a hot stove nor put in hot water, or the blood will again become hardened.

4. The vessel used for the purpose of soaking meat may not be used for the preparation of any other food.

5. After the meat has been soaked, some of the water must be allowed to drain off, so that the salt may not dissolve at once and become ineffective in drawing out the blood. Further, the meat should not be allowed to completely dry, for then the salt would not adhere to it at all and would fail to drain the blood from it.

6. Every square inch of the meat or poultry should be salted.

7. The salt should be coarser than flour so that it may not dissolve too quickly, and yet not too coarse for then it would entirely drop from the meat.

8. The meat that has been salted must be placed where the blood can easily drain off.

9. The meat should remain in the salt for one whole hour.

10. After the meat has been salted for the proper length of time, the salt should be thoroughly shaken off and the meat is to be washed again three times.

11. Eggs found in poultry, no matter what their stage of development, must be soaked, salted, and purged as if they were meat.

12. Meat that remains unsoaked and unsalted for three full days after the animal has been ritually slaughtered may not be used.

13. The law of Moses as found in Genesis 32:33 forbids the use of the hindquarter part of even "clean" animals, unless the forbidden parts and blood vessels are properly removed. Most butchers know how to purge only the forequarter of kosher animals. Therefore, orthodox Jews generally use the forequarter of meat only and abstain from using the hindquarter.

14. Meat and dairy products may not be eaten or boiled together. It is customary to mark all utensils used for dairy foods, so that they may not be interchanged with those used for meat. Further, after eating meat, or even a dish prepared with meat, one should wait six hours before eating dairy food.[12]

Although blood can be drained from the arteries, as in the above mentioned process, it is impossible to remove blood from the capillaries. This could therefore be understood as an ultimate prohibition against any consumption of flesh. Still, even if one considers the process of koshering to be legitimate, it is an obvious burden placed upon the Jewish people, perhaps in the hope that they will eventually give up flesh-foods altogether. If eating meat is such a detailed, long, and drawn-out process, why not give it up entirely?

To summarize, blood is adamantly proscribed in the Old Testament. In order to get around these restrictions and give meat-eating some divine basis, the koshering laws have been developed within the biblical and rabbinical traditions. Still, the whole koshering process does not accomplish its end; although liquid blood may be drained to some extent, the blood remains in the flesh in solidified form. Thus, even though some persons are attracted to the eating of meat, seafood, eggs, and other things produced by semen and blood and eaten in the form of dead bodies, God, in the scriptures, tries to discourage such a diet. There is encouragement in biblical texts to use free will to develop one's spirituality by showing compassion and concern for all of God's creation.

An example of such compassion can be seen on Yom Kippur, the Day of Atonement, when all observant Jews practice austerity of the tongue (by fasting) and try to evoke God's compassion by prayer and contemplation. On that day, no leather shoes are allowed in the synagogue. The reason, it has been pointed out, is the hypocrisy of asking God for mercy and compassion while showing a lack of the same toward our fellow creatures.

Another example of spiritual compassion in the Jewish tradition can be seen in the story of Daniel. The Bible records that he and his three comrades were held captive by King Nebuchadnezzar of Babylon. The king had sent his servant to Daniel with rich foods, including meat and wine. Daniel said to the servant that he and his friends would not take the meat or drink the wine. "But the king only wants you to be strong and healthy," said the servant. Daniel then replied, "Then bring me and my comrades vegetables and water. Try it for ten days and then see for yourself if we are not stronger and wiser than the others who eat the king's food."

"All right," said the king's servant. "I will try this for ten days—but if you are not stronger and wiser, the king may take my life."

For ten days, the four men ate vegetables and drank water. Then the king's servant looked at them. "You do look healthier and stronger," he said. "It is hard to believe. From now on, I will give you only vegetables and water." (Daniel 1:3-21) This is the same Daniel who, thrown into a lion's den, came out unharmed, perhaps because the animal sensed the vegetarian saint's extreme compassion and lack of ill will.

Today a much larger proportion of Jewish people share Daniel's vegetarianism than do their neighbors. The North American Jewish Vegetarian Society propounds the meatless ideal, as does the London-based International Jewish Vegetarian Society. Both are gaining enthusiastic supporters at a modest but steady rate. In Israel there have been three vegetarian chief rabbis in twenty-five years and over four percent of the population is vegetarian—and the numbers keep increasing. Israel, in fact, has the largest concentration of religious vegetarians in the world, with the obvious exception of India.

East Indians, it should be noted, have traditionally referred to Western culture by the Sanskrit word *mleccha,* indicating the West's predilection toward meat-eating and other less savory characteristics. Interestingly, the Hebrew *m'leecha,* pronounced much the same way, is the word which describes the whole koshering phenomenon. The connection between these two words must have come as no surprise to the early Hebrews, for their own word for "meat" (*basar*) was explained by the Talmudists as being composed of the initials *bet* ("shame"), *sin* ("corruption") and *resh* ("worms"). The word as a whole, then, was to be reminiscent of the well-known quotation from the Talmud *(Aboth, perek* 2, *mishna* 7): "The more flesh, the more worms"—a discouragement against gluttony.

Another command against gluttony comes from the Hebrew sage Ramban, who, commenting on the Biblical imperative to "be holy" (Lev. 19:2), admonishes the Jewish people: "Be holy by abstaining from those things which are permitted to you....For those who drink wine and eat meat all the time are considered 'scoundrels with a Torah license'."[13]

Indeed, Judaism exhorts its followers not to be gluttons but to be modest and refined, to bring in a new era of God-fearing people who abide by the laws and covenants of Moses and Abraham. Jews must, by righteous behavior, secure their place in the world to come. And they must make this world as spiritual a place as possible, in preparation for the coming of the messiah. The time of the messiah, so tradition holds, will be a time when peace, compassion and mercy will reign supreme: "For behold, I create new heavens and a new earth, and the former shall not be remembered—and they shall plant vineyards and eat the fruit of them—the wolf and the lamb shall feed together and the lion shall eat straw like the bullock. They shall not hurt nor destroy in all My holy mountain." (Isaiah 65:17, 25)

It may be thought that the Jewish tradition will not allow this prophecy to unfold, that it has strayed too far from the purity of such visionary compassion. Change will be difficult, to be sure. Apart from habit and tradition, custom has dictated for centuries that the able Jewish family must provide expensive meats and fish as delicacies for the Sabbath.

However, a close study of the Hebrew scriptures reveals that one need not eat meat on the Sabbath.[14] In fact, if it is offensive to a particular individual, say the scriptures, then one must indeed *avoid* meat on the Sabbath.[15] Further, it should be known that the Talmud (*Pessachim* 109a) states, "Rabbi Yehuda, who said that there is no piety on the Sabbath unless one eats meat, agrees that this only applied at the time when the Temple of Sacrifice, in Jerusalem, was in existence."

It is further stated in the Talmud (*Tracte Babba Bathra* 608) by Rabbi Yishmael, "From the day that the holy Temple was destroyed, it would have been right to have imposed upon ourselves the law prohibiting the eating of flesh. But the rabbis have laid down a wise and logical ruling that the authorities must not impose any decree unless the majority of the members of the community are able to abide by it. Otherwise the law and those who administer it get into disrepute." The laws in regard to meat-eating, then, were developed by the early rabbis to avoid losing followers. It was an emergency measure that was meant to insure the survival of the Jewish tradition.

REFERENCES

1. Richard Schwartz, *Judaism and Vegetarianism* (New York, Exposition Press, 1982), p. 70.
2. Rabbi Samuel H. Dresner, *The Jewish Dietary Laws* (New York, The Rabbinical Assembly of America, 1982), p. 25.
3. Ibid. p. 32.
4. See Ben Isaacson, *Dictionary of the Jewish Religion*, ed. David C. Gross (New York, Bantam Books, 1979), p. 54.
5. Rabbi James M. Labeau, *The Jewish Dietary Laws: Sanctify Life* (New York, The United Synagogue of America, 1983), p. 71.
6. Richard Schwartz, "Vegetarianism from a Jewish Vegetarian's Perspective," *The Journal of Halacha and Contemporary Society*, Spring, 1982, Vol. II, No. I, p. 85.
7. *The Slaughter of Food Animals*, a brochure by The Royal Society for the Prevention of Cruelty to Animals (RSPCA), England, 1985, p. 10.
8. *Ibid.* p. 12.
9. Roberta Kalechofsky, *Haggadah for the Liberated Lamb* (Mass., Micah Pub., 1985), p. 8.
10. *Ibid.*
11. *Ibid.*
12. Hyman E. Golden, *A Jew and His Duties* (New York, Hebrew Pub. Co., 1953), p. 68.
13. Rabbi Alfred S. Cohen, senior editor, "Vegetarianism from a Jewish Perspective," *The Journal of Halacha and Contemporary Society*, Fall, 1981, Vol. 1, No. 2, p. 50.
14. *Ibid.* pp. 40-41.
15. *Ibid.*

ISLAM

Chapter 4

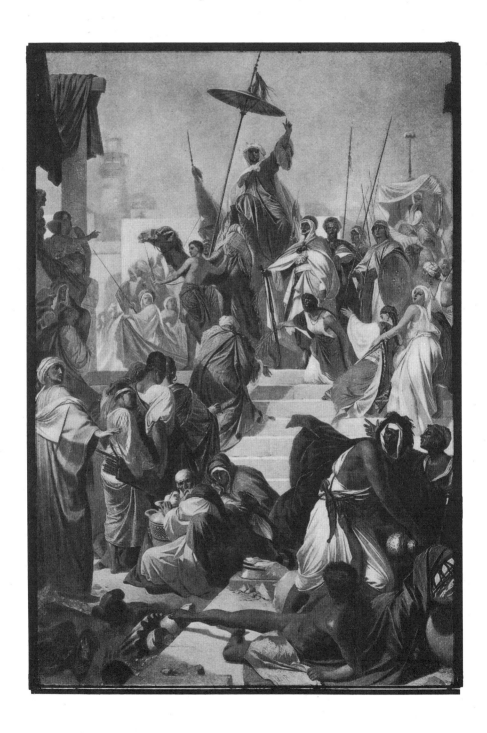

ISLAM

*"Whoever is kind to the creatures of God
is kind to himself."*

—Hadith of Prophet Mohammed

The Islamic tradition holds that in Mecca, the birthplace of Mohammed, no creature be slaughtered and that perfect harmony exist between all living things. In fact, Muslim pilgrims approach Mecca wearing a shroud (*ihram*), and from the time they don this religious apparel, absolutely no killing is allowed: not mosquitoes, lice, grasshoppers, or any other living creature. If a pilgrim sees an insect on the ground, he will gesture to stop his comrades from inadvertently stepping on it. Thus, while Islam is not generally viewed as a religion that endorses vegetarianism and kindness to animals, the Islamic tradition does have a great deal to say about a person's relationship to the animal world.

Islam, it may be noted, is considered a relatively new religion. Although its own tradition holds that Islamic principles can be traced back to Adam, the religion was actually founded by the prophet Mohammed in the early seventh century. And even though the Islamic faith considers it meritorious to perish in battle on its behalf, it also reveres the prophet Mohammed's words concerning compassion and nonviolence—especially toward animals.

The Example of Mohammed

Biographies of Mohammed include narrations that clearly depict his love for animals. And while one would be hard-pressed to find Muslims

59

today who feel that their religion supports vegetarianism (although there are certain sects that do), Mohammed's teachings in this regard are clear. For instance, Margoliouth, one of Mohammed's chief biographers, writes, "His humanity extended itself to the lower creation. He forbade the employment of towing birds as targets for marksmen and remonstrated with those who ill-treated their camels. When some of his followers had set fire to an ant-hill," Margoliouth continues, "he compelled them to extinguish it....Acts of cruelty were swept away by him."[1]

Other biographers, such as Dr. M. Hafiz Syed, point out that Mohammed instructed those who eat meat to wash out their mouth before going to pray. While it is certainly a Muslim custom to clean one's mouth before going to prayer, many biographers say that only meat is emphasized in this connection and not any other food.[2] To a vegetarian Muslim, this would come as no surprise.

Why, it may be asked, did Mohammed allow meat-eating at all? One possible answer is that, because he based much of his teaching on the Old Testament, Mohammed employed the same concession for meat-eaters as God did in the biblical scriptures and the same techniques of gradualism. Although total compassion and abstinence from killing were the ideal, Mohammed had to bring his followers to that platform slowly so as not to repel potential adherents (who were not ready for that particular level of spiritual understanding).

Mohammed knew his people well. Before the advent of Islam, the people of Arabia embraced a plurality of gods, bigamy was the rule, and drunkenness the norm. If a man's wife gave birth to a baby girl, the couple out of shame would bury her alive (Koran, surah 6, verse 140). Sexual relations between mothers and sons were so widespread that the Koran contained prohibitions (Koran, surah 4, verses 19-24). It was Mohammed's mission to uplift his people, but the Prophet knew that radical change was doomed to failure. Like the great religious reformers before him, Mohammed considered the time, place and circumstances surrounding his mission. In fact, Mohammed openly admitted that he only taught men according to their mental capacities: "...for if you speak all things to all men—some will not understand."[3]

All esoteric teachings are revealed on two levels, one for the average person and one for those who are more spiritually evolved. In this regard, Mohammed said, "The teachings were sent in seven dialects; and in every one of its sentences there is an external and an internal meaning....I received two kinds of knowledge: one of these I taught—but if I had taught them the other, it would have broken their throats."[4] Although Islamic tradition and Arabic linguists have long since developed an explanation for the peculiar expression "broken their throats," many vegetarian Muslims have suggested that vegetarianism is implied with this phrase.

In fact, Mohammed could only have been in favor of vegetarianism, although he may have been unable to impose this philosophy on the majority. He always showed the greatest compassion—"universal compassion"— and he exhorted his followers to do the same. A touching example from Mohammed's life shows how far his empathy extended. Awaking from a nap one afternoon, he found a small, sick cat fast asleep on the edge of his cloak. The Prophet cut off his garment so that the cat could sleep undisturbed. Is this a man who would advocate the unnecessary slaughter of harmless beasts? "Show sympathy to others," Mohammed taught, "especially to those who are weaker than you."[5]

In one popular tradition (Hadith), Mohammed is depicted as having rebuked his followers for not showing universal compassion. "But we do show compassion," they insisted, "—to our wives, children and relatives." The Prophet responded, "It is not this to which I refer. I am speaking of universal mercy."

One advantage of Islam's being a newer religion is that many specific facts concerning Mohammed's diet and attitude toward animals are freshly remembered and preserved. The Prophet's earliest biographers indicate that he preferred vegetarian foods, saying that he liked milk diluted with water, yogurt with butter or nuts, and cucumbers with dates. His favorite fruits, which he was known to subsist on for weeks at a time, were pomegranates, grapes and figs, and he liked a morning drink of soaked, crushed dates. He was particularly fond of honey, often eating it mixed with vinegar, and he is quoted as saying that in a house where there is vinegar and honey, there will certainly be the blessings of the Lord. He also liked a preparation then called *hees,* made from butter, dates and yogurt. According to extensive biographical accounts, furthermore, Mohammed has been quoted as saying, "Where there is an abundance of vegetables, hosts of angels will descend on that place."

Not everyone, Mohammed knew, could be expected to follow such strict dietary habits. And the Koran, like the Bible, offers concessions as intermediary stages toward a pure and spiritual diet: "O ye who believe! Eat of the good things with which we have supplied you, and give God thanks if ye are His worshippers. Only that which dieth of itself, blood, and swine's flesh, and that over which any other name than that of God's has been invoked, hath God forbidden you." (Koran, surah 5, verse 1) Here the Koran clearly states that pork is impure and that animal blood is not fit for human consumption (a legacy from the Old Testament). The Muslims, then, run into the same dietary contradiction as the Jews: blood is forbidden—it is impossible to completely separate blood from animal flesh—so if one eats meat, blood is being consumed as well. In the words of the Koran, this, indeed, is a "portent for people who think."

The Koran goes on to say that if one needs to eat forbidden foods to stay alive, that is no sin. But this was hardly the case for Arabs living in a world that offered a great variety of alternatives to meat. They had olives and apples from Syria, raisins from Israel, wheat from Egypt, millet from southern Arabia, rice from the valley of the Jordan and from India, where they also procured spices.[6] If this concession did not apply in early times, it carries even less weight now, with the convenience of modern transportation making foods from all over the world accessible.

Mohammed's death underlined the place of vegetarianism in Islam. The story goes that a non-Muslim woman invited Mohammed and some of his companions to a meal and served them poisoned meat. The Prophet knew by spiritual insight that the meat was poisoned, for he alone ate it, ordering his companions not to do so. Although it was not his custom to eat meat, or any other food prepared by a non-Muslim, on this occasion, mysteriously, he did. The poisoned meat put him in a sickbed for about two years, and finally, in A.D. 632, he died. According to some scholars, Mohammed ate the poisoned meat just to show the stubborn masses the harmfulness of meat-eating.

The Koran, moreover, contains several references pertinent to vegetarianism, such as the following (which are similar to and apparently based upon Genesis 1:29):

> Let man reflect on the food he eats: how we poured out the rain abundantly, and split the earth into fissures, and how we then made the grains to grow, and vines and reeds, olives and palms and gardens and fruits and pastures—an enjoyment for you and your cattle to delight in.

The following verses continue on the same theme:

> It is God who sends down water out of the sky, and with it quickens the earth after it is dead. Surely, in that is a sign for people who have ears to hear. In cattle, too, there is a lesson for you: we give you to drink of what is in their bellies, between filth and blood—pure milk, sweet to those who drink. And we give you the fruits of the palms and the vines from which you derive sweet-tasting liquid and fair provision. Indeed, this is a sign for men of understanding. And your Lord inspires the bees, saying, "Build your homes in the mountains, in the trees and in the thatch of roots, then feed on every kind of fruit and follow the ways of your Lord,

so easy to go upon." Then there comes forth out of their bellies a liquid of various colors wherein is healing for men. Truly, in this is a sign for people who reflect. (Koran, surah 16, verses 65-69)

Ultimately, the Koran encourages Muslims to eat wholesome, healthful foods. In describing lawful and unlawful foods, the Koran emphasizes that "He [the Prophet] makes lawful to them the good things of life and he forbids them the bad things." (Koran, surah 7, verse 157) The implications of this teaching are brought out even more clearly by Al-Ghazzali (1058-1111), one of Islam's most brilliant philosophers, who wrote in his book *Ihya Ulum ul-Din*, "Eating the meat of a cow causes disease (*marz*), its milk is health (*safa*) and its clarified butter (*ghee*) is medicine (*dava*). Compassionate eating leads to compassionate living."[7]

The Koran clearly evokes compassion and mercy toward animals, and although many Muslims never consider vegetarianism, certain sects, such as the Shiites, do have a core of vegetarian followers. Islamic mystics, such as the Sufis, also hold vegetarianism as a high spiritual ideal.

The Sufi Tradition

There is an ancient story about a woman Sufi saint, Hazrat Rabia Basri, who would regularly go to a particular mountain in the forest in order to meditate in perfect tranquility. When she would go, all the animals of the forest would come near to enjoy her good company. One day, another Sufi arrived. But as soon as he approached, all the animals ran away, as if in fear. Completely vexed, the Sufi inquired of Rabia Basri, "Why do the animals run?"

Rabia countered with another question: "What have you eaten today?" The Sufi confessed that he had eaten an onion fried in some fat. The wise Sufi woman concluded, "You eat their fat! Why should they not flee from you?" This famous Sufi tale is perhaps indicative of the Islamic mystical perspective on human-animal interrelations.

A great contemporary Sufi master, Muhammad Rahim Bawa Muhaiyaddeen, tells another parable entitled "The Hunter Learns Compassion from the Fawn." Presented in the Sufi oral tradition and in the ancient Tamil language, this story conveys, with a simple illustration, the all-encompassing compassion ideally sought by all religionists. It was originally told for the benefit of a small group of children, but its truth extends beyond any age group. The tale was preserved in a book entitled *Come to the Secret Garden* and is reproduced as follows:

...Once there was a man who liked to go hunting. He would go into the forest carrying a gun or a bow and arrow, and he would shoot deer, elk, and other animals. Like most hunters he enjoyed eating all the animals he killed, but he found deer meat especially tasty.

Now this man had been hunting, killing, and eating like this for most of his life. Then one day he came upon a deer giving milk to her fawn. This made him happy because he was tired, and he knew that the deer could not run away while her baby was nursing. So he shot her. But before dying, the deer cried, 'O man, you have shot me, so go ahead and eat me, but do not harm my child! Let it live and go free!'

'I understand what you are asking,' the hunter replied, 'but I plan to take your child home, raise it, and make it nice and fat. Then one day it too will become meat for me to eat.'

The little fawn heard this and said, 'O man are such thoughts acceptable to God?'

The hunter laughed. 'God created animals for men to kill and eat.'

'O man, you are right. God did create some beings so that others could eat them. But what about you? If there is a law like that for us, then perhaps there is also such a law for you. Think about it. There is only one person ready to eat me, but there are so many eagerly waiting to eat you. Don't you know that? Someday in the very presence of God Himself, grubs, worms, the tiny insects of hell, and even the earth itself will be quite happy to devour you. You who are a human being must think about this. When we deer are killed, we are eaten right away, but when you die you will be consumed in hell ever so slowly, over a long period of time. You will be subjected to hell in so many rebirths.

'O man, God created me and He created you. You are a man. God created you from earth, fire, water, air and ether. I am an animal, but God created me from these same elements. You walk on two legs, I walk on four. Even though our skin and color are different, our flesh is the same. Think about the many ways in which we are alike.

'If someone had killed your mother while you were nursing, how would you feel? Most men would feel sorry if they killed a deer with her fawn. They would cry, "Oh, I didn't know!" But you don't seem to have any compassion. You are a murderer. You have killed so many lives, but you never stop to think how sad you would be if someone killed your mother. Instead you are happy to kill not only my mother, but you also want to kill me and eat me. Since you are a human being, you should think about this. Even the cruelest and most demonic of beasts would stop to think about what I have said.

'Can't you understand the sadness of a child whose mother has just been killed? What you said to my mother and to me is terrible and has caused me great pain. O man, you have neither God's compassion nor human compassion. You do not even have a human conscience. All your life you have been drinking the blood and eating the flesh of animals without realizing what you have been doing. You love flesh and enjoy murder. If you had a conscience or any sense of justice, if you were born as a true human being, you would think about this. God is looking at me and at you...'

'Little fawn, everything you have said is true,' the hunter admitted. Then he gently picked up the body of the mother and led the baby deer home.

That night he told the other hunters what the baby deer had taught him. All who heard the story cried. 'So often we have eaten deer meat, but now that you have told us this, we see the karma that has come to us through the food we enjoyed. Our bodies are in a state of turmoil. We realize now that we had no compassion or wisdom.' And they all decided to stop eating such food.

'Let the baby deer go,' one man said. 'No, give me the deer,' said another. 'I will raise it until it grows up and then I will set it free.'

But the hunter decided to raise the fawn by himself. And over the years that deer showed him more love than his own children did. 'This gentle being is capable of more love and gratitude than a human being,' the man thought. 'It kisses and licks me and makes contented sounds when I feed it. And it even sleeps at my feet.'

So the years passed until the deer was fully grown. Then one day the man took it into the forest and set it free.

My children, each of us must be aware of everything we do. All young animals have love and compassion. And if we remember that every creation was young once, we will never kill another life. We will not harm or attack any living creature...[8]

The story represents a clearly vegetarian tradition within Islamic mysticism. This same tradition explains *qurban,* the animal slaughtering process ordained for Muslims, as having an esoteric as well as its usual exoteric meaning. While *qurban* externally refers only to Muslim dietary laws, which are similar to those of the Jews, inwardly *qurban* requires that we sacrifice our life to the devotion and service of God, and that we sacrifice our beastly qualities instead of the life of an animal. "*Qurban* is not slaughtering chickens and cows and goats," explains Bawa Muhaiyaddeen. "There are four hundred trillion, ten thousand beasts here in the heart which must be slaughtered. They must be slaughtered in the *qalb* [the inner heart]. After these things have been slaughtered, what is eaten can then be distinguished as either *halal* [permissible] or *haraam* [forbidden]." Ultimately, the Sufi master concludes, "everything that is seen in the world is *haraam.* What is seen in Allah [God] alone is *halaal.* Please eat that."[9]

Still, even in the traditional *qurban,* the prayer known as the *kalimah*[10] is recited to remove the baser qualities of the animal. According to the Sufi tradition, the recitation of the powerful Third Kalimah will not only purify the animal slaughtered for consumption, but also all those involved with the sacrifice, so that they will no longer want to slaughter animals. This will only work, however, if the prayer is said with pure devotion.

As in Judaism, sacrificial animal slaughter is a detailed process for Muslims. And the whole procedure, again, is meant to minimize the killing of animals. In the words of Bawa Muhaiyaddeen:

> While you recite the *Kalimah,* you must complete the severing in three strokes of the knife, one for each recitation. The knife has to be swept around three times, and it must not touch the bone. It must be extremely sharp, and the length is prescribed according to each animal—so much for a fowl, so much for a goat, so much for a cow....Also, the animal must not regurgitate any food, and it must not make any noise; otherwise, it becomes *haraam.*
>
> The person who holds the animal and the person who cuts it must always observe the five times prayer. Therefore, it must be the *Imam* and the *mu'azzin* who perform the *qurban,* because very often they are the only ones who regularly observe the five times prayer. This also means that the *qurban* must take place near a mosque where two such people can always be found. Before beginning the slaughter, they must first perform their ablutions, and then they must recite the *kalimah* three times and feed water to the animal which is to be sacrificed. The neck of the animal must be turned in the direction of the *Qiblah* [in other words, the animal must be pointed in the direction of the holy: for Muslims it is Mecca], so that the eyes of the sacrificial animal look into the eyes of the person who is doing the sacrifice. The person must look into the eyes of the animal and then, saying the *kalimah,* he must cut the neck. And he must continue to look into the eyes of the animal until its soul departs, repeating the *Zikr* all the while. Then after the soul has departed, he must say the *kalimah* once again and wash the knife. Only then can he move on to the next animal. He has to look into the animal's eyes, he has to watch the tears of the animal, and he has to watch the animal's eyes until it dies—hopefully, his heart will change.[11]

Muhaiyaddeen goes on to narrate a Sufi tradition further supporting the vegetarian perspective:

> Allah told Muhammad, 'With this qurban the killing will be greatly reduced, for where they used to kill 1,000 or 2,000 in one day, they will now be able to slaughter only ten or fifteen animals. If they started after morning prayers, it would be ten o'clock by the time they are ready to begin, and they could slaughter only until eleven o'clock, when they must prepare for

the next prayer. In addition, it takes about fifteen or twenty minutes for each animal, because he has to wait until the soul has departed.' This is how Allah instructed the Prophet.

Then the people complained, 'How can we do this? We can cut only so few! Our enjoyments and our festivals are being curtailed.'

But Allah said, 'Each one of you does not need to sacrifice one animal; you do not need to sacrifice one animal for each family. In place of forty fowls, kill one goat. In place of forty goats, kill ten cows. And in place of forty cows, kill ten camels. Sacrifice ten camels and then share the meat among the different families.' So in place of four hundred animals only forty might be killed. The killing was reduced by that much. Thus, Allah passed down the commands to the Prophet to reduce the taking of lives.[12]

Muhaiyaddeen concludes, "If you understand the qurban from within with wisdom, its purpose is to reduce this killing. But if you look at it from outside, it is meant to supply desire with food, to supply the craving of the base desires..."[13] Thus, the esoteric imperative behind Islamic dietary laws is that Muslims aspire after compassion and mercy, first by minimizing the amount of animals one is able to kill (by following all the regulations), and then, it is to be hoped, by giving it up altogether.

The Koran, interestingly, lists forbidden rather than permitted foods. And its concern is always with meat. This encouraged Middle Eastern scholar Michael Cook, in his book *Muhammed*, to write, "Vegetarians have no problem [with Koranic dietary laws]."[14] Scriptural food laws, then, appear to be a deliberate burden upon meat-eating believers. They, and not their vegetarian brothers, must observe very strict dietary laws that serve only to curtail a flesh-eating regimen.

Compassion and Mercy

The Koran itself exalts total compassion and mercy. In fact, all of the Koran's 114 chapters, with the exception of one, begin Bismillahir-rahmanir-rahim, that is, "Allah is merciful and compassionate." It should be noted, furthermore, that the name for God used most frequently in the Koran is al-Rahim, which means "the All Compassionate." The next most frequent name is al-Raham—"the All-merciful." Elsewhere, the Koran describes God as Arham al-Rahimin, "the Most Merciful of the Merciful." The emphasis throughout is on the all-encompassing nature of God's mercy. A lack of mercy toward lower creatures would be inconsistent with that all-encompassing nature. Mohammed, as we have shown, demonstrated such mercy in his own life. An indication that one is a true follower might therefore be to emulate Mohammed by observing similar compassion and mercy. Vegetarianism would be a tangible step in that direction.

If we base our conception of Islam on the Koran, the Islamic mystical tradition, and especially on Mohammed's life and teachings, we find that vegetarianism and kindness toward animals are of central importance—this we have shown and hope to reinforce with the following quotations. These are well-known translations from the Arabic *Hadith* (literally "traditions," texts as authoritative as the Koran), compiled by the Islamic scholar M. Hafiz Syed:

> The Prophet passed by certain people who were shooting arrows at a ram, and hated that, saying, "Maim not the brute beasts."

> The Prophet, seen wiping the face of his horse with his wrapper, and being questioned in regard to it, said, "At night I received a reprimand from God in regard to my horse."

> A man once robbed some eggs from the nest of a bird, whereupon the Prophet had them restored to the nest. "Fear God in these dumb animals," said the Prophet, "and ride them when they are fit to be ridden—and get off them when they are tired."

> "Verily, are there rewards for our doing good to quadrupeds and giving them water to drink?" asked the disciples. And the Prophet answered, "There are rewards for benefiting every animal having a moist liver." [i.e. everyone alive!][15]

Popular Islam, like other contemporary forms of the world's great religions, does not overtly speak in favor of vegetarianism. It is ultimately up to each individual to decide whether he or she will adopt the principle of kindness to animals. The scriptures certainly do not demand that we slaughter, or support the slaughter, of defenseless beings, and there is sufficient evidence that the highest religious truth is to cherish all life and emulate God's all-encompassing love and compassion. In light of the above Hadith, commonly attributed to Mohammed, the reader is encouraged to decide for himself or herself as to whether the compassion of the Prophet, and that of the Koran, extends to animals.

REFERENCES

1. Quoted in Rev. V. A. Holmes-Gore, *These We Have Not Loved* (London, The C. W. Daniel Co., Ltd., 1946), pp. 6-7.
2. M. Hafiz Syed, *Thus Spoke Muhammed* (Madras, Amra Press, 1962), p. 6.
3. *Ibid.,* p. 8.
4. Quoted in Nadarbeg K. Mizra, "The Sayings of Mohammed," *Reincarnation and Islam* (Madras, 1927), pp. 4-5.
5. Bilkiz Alladin, *The Story of Mohammed The Prophet* (India, Hemkunt Press, 1979), pp. 12-13.
6. Reay Tannahill, *Food in History* (New York, Stein and Day Pub., 1973), p. 174.
7. *A Review of Beef in Ancient India* (India, Gita Press, 1971), p. 167.
8. M. R. Bawa Muhaiyaddeen, *Come to the Secret Garden* (Philadelphia, PA., The Fellowship Press, 1985), pp. 24-28.
9. M. R. Bawa Muhaiyaddeen, *Asma' ul-Husna: The 99 Beautiful Names of Allah* (PA, The Fellowship Press, 1979), p. 181.
10. *Kalimah* is a general Islamic prayer considered especially purifying when used to sanctify the slaughtering of a food animal in the Muslim tradition. In the Hindu tradition, however, Kali Ma refers to a goddess whose followers thrive on offering blood sacrifices to her. It is considered by Puranic Hinduism to be an inferior form of worship.
11. M. R. Bawa Muhaiyaddeen, *Asma' ul-Husna: The 99 Beautiful Names of Allah* (Philadelphia, PA, The Fellowship Press, 1979), p. 182.
12. *Ibid.*
13. *Ibid.,* p. 183.
14. Michael Cook, *Muhammed* (England, Oxford University Press, 1983) p. 65.
15. M. Hafiz Syed, *op. cit.,* pp. 10-20.

AHIMSA AND EASTERN RELIGION

Chapter 5

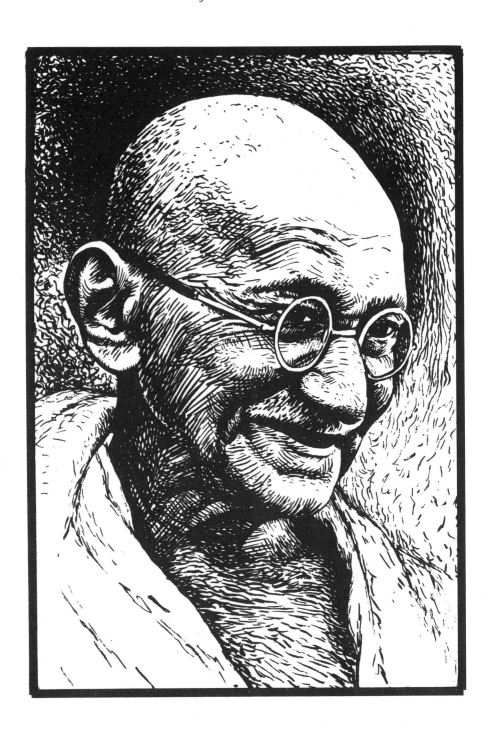

AHIMSA AND EASTERN RELIGION

"Ahimsa is the highest duty."

—Padma Purana 1.31.27

The doctrine of *ahimsa* (noninjury to sentient beings) was originally enunciated in the Vedas, India's ancient Sanskrit scriptures. *Ahimsa* is integral to most Eastern religions, which view it as one of their most important religious doctrines—and vegetarianism as its fundamental extension.

To understand *ahimsa* and its role in the religious life of the East, it is helpful to understand the scriptures that describe it and the tradition that gave it life. There is some controversy concerning just when the Vedas were compiled. Tradition, however, ascribes a date of around 3,000 B.C., a position shared by Arnold Toynbee and other sympathetic purveyors of Eastern religions. Prior to their written form, the Vedas were transmitted orally from master to disciple, reaching back, says the tradition, to a time before the created universe.

Vedic literature was written in Sanskrit, ancestor of the Indo-European languages such as Latin, Greek, German and English. These Sanskrit texts are vast in size. The *Rig Veda* alone contains 1,017 hymns; the *Mahabharata* (which includes the famed *Bhagavad Gita*) consists of 110,000 couplets; the Puranas, or Vedic histories, contain hundreds of thousands of verses; and there are 108 Upanishads, texts that summarize the philosophical teachings of the Vedas.

Most remarkable about these writings is their continuing impact on contemporary world cultures. Far from obsolete, the teachings of the Vedas animate the social, ethical, philosophical and religious lives of millions of

73

people around the world. Even such modern-day peace initiatives as Gandhi's nonviolent movement in India and Dr. Martin Luther King's freedom marches in the United States took their inspiration from the Vedic principle of *ahimsa*.

Ahimsa loosely translates as "nonviolence." In the Vedic tradition, however, the word possesses a much broader meaning: "Having no ill feeling for any living being, in all manners possible and for all times, is called *ahimsa*, and it should be the desired goal of all seekers." (*Patanjali Yoga Sutras*, 2.30)

Later Pali manuscripts, too, promote *ahimsa*, qualifying that it be accompanied by camaraderie (*mettacitta*),[1] freedom from anger (*avera*)[2] and an aversion to ill will (*abyapajja*).[3] *Ahimsa* further requires that one not utter words that are either harsh (*akakkasa*)[4] or hurting (*na abhisajjana*).[5] By this definition, *ahimsa* includes subtle as well as overt forms of nonviolence.

The *Manusmriti*, one of India's most renowned sacred texts, says: "Without the killing of living beings, meat cannot be made available, and since killing is contrary to the principles of *ahimsa*, one must give up eating meat."[6]

The Vedic tradition condemns more, however, than just those who eat meat. Equally guilty, it says, is anyone assisting in animal slaughter, sanctioning it, anyone who cuts the flesh, buys, sells, or even serves it.[7] Only those who have not participated in any of these activities can be considered true practitioners of *ahimsa*.

Zoroastrianism, Sikhism and Jainism

Among the less prominent Eastern religions that practice true *ahimsa* is Zoroastrianism (also known as Magianism, Mazdaism or Parseeism). Originally a sect that flourished in ancient Persia, it is now centered primarily in Bombay. Zarathushtra (Zoroaster in Greek), who founded this religion, was an ardent and well-known advocate of vegetarianism in Persia around 600 B.C. Under Islamic rule, many Zoroastrians fled from Iran in the seventh century A.D., and their modern successors are the Parsees of India. There is a strong adherence to the vegetarian way of life by the 200,000 Zoroastrians left in the world today.

Sikhism, founded by Guru Nanak (1469-1538), is an interesting blend of Hindu and Islamic beliefs. Because of the Muslim influence, most branches of the Sikh religion are not strictly vegetarian. Still, according to Sikh scholar Swaran Singh Sanehi of the Academy of Namdhari culture: "Sikh scriptures support vegetarianism fully. Sikhs from the period of Guru

Nanak had adopted the Hindu tradition and way of living in many ways. Their disliking for flesh-foods was also a part of the same tradition and way of living. Guru Nanak considered meat-eating improper—particularly for those who are trying to meditate."[8] Of the ten million Sikhs, the Namdhari sect and Yogi Bhajan's 3HO Golden Temple Movement are strictly vegetarian.

Jainism is an Eastern religion whose cardinal teaching is *ahimsa*.. Unlike the Zoroastrians and Sikhs, Jains have remained faithful to *ahimsa* throughout their history. Continuing with their preceptor Mahavira (599-527 B.C.), Jainism has grown very strong and today boasts four million followers, all of whom are strict vegetarians. In India, they are famous for their "animal hospitals," and it was a Jain monk, Hiravijaya-Suri, who persuaded the Muslim emperor Akbar (1556-1605) to prohibit the killing of animals on certain days.[9] Akbar himself eventually renounced hunting and fully adopted the vegetarian ideal, although it is sometimes said that he was not strict in his non-meat-eating resolve.[10]

Universal Ahimsa

All life should be revered, say the Vedas, for the body is merely an outer shell for the spirit within. This is the philosophical thread that runs through nearly all Eastern religions. Still, the Vedic literature acknowledges that certain bodies are more highly evolved than others, as described in the following verses:

> Animate beings (*jiva*) are better than inanimate beings (*ajiva*); breathing creatures (*prana-bhrit*) are best among the animate ones; among breathing beings, those who possess a mind (*sa-chitta*) are the best. Among those equipped with a mind, the creatures who have sensorial experiences (*indriyavritti*) are the best. Those experiencing taste (*rasa-vedin*) are better than those who experience only touch (*sparsa-vedin*). Those who experience smell (*gandha-vid*) are better than the above two. Those who experience sound (*shabda-vid*) are better than the above three. Those who know the difference in the various types of colors (*rupa-veda-vid*) are better than those above. Those having teeth on both sides of the mouth are still better. Among these, again, the best are those who have many feet (*bahu-pada*). Four-footed ones are still better. Two-footed ones are better than the four-footed ones. The beings belonging to the four castes (*chatur-varna*) [i.e. human beings] are better than other two-footed creatures. Among the four castes, the intellectuals and priests (*brahmanas*) are the best. Among the *brahmanas*, those well-versed in the Vedas are best.

Among these, again, the best are those who know the implications (*artha*) of the Vedas. Still better are those who can dispel doubts (*samshaya-cchetta*). Among these, again, those are the best who perform their own duties. Even more excellent are those who are free from attachment (*mukta-sanga*) and do not hanker after the fruit of their own merit (*bhakta*). These are known as the devotees of God. (*Shrimad Bhagavatam* 3.29.28-32)

According to the Sanskrit Vedic literature, there are 8,400,000 different species of life, and although some are unquestionably more advanced than others, to treat any one of them in a disrespectful or harmful way is a violation of *ahimsa*.

REFERENCES

1. Unto Tahtinen, *Ahimsa: Nonviolence in Indian Tradition* (London, Rider and Co., 1976), p. 11.
2. *Ibid.*
3. *Ibid.*
4. *Ibid.*
5. *Ibid.*
6. *Manusmriti* 5.48.
7. *Ibid.*,5.51.
8. Swaran Singh Sanehi, *Vegetarianism in Sikhism* (Madras, The Vegetarian Way, 1977), p. 34.
9. Padmanabh S. Jaini, *The Jain Path of Purification* (Berkeley, University of California Press, 1979), p. 284.
10. Christopher Chapple, "Noninjury to Animals: Jain and Buddhist Perspectives," in *Animal Sacrifices: Religious Perspectives on the Use of Animals in Science*, ed. Tom Regan, (Philadelphia, PA, Temple Univ. Press, 1986), p. 217.

BUDDHISM
Chapter 6

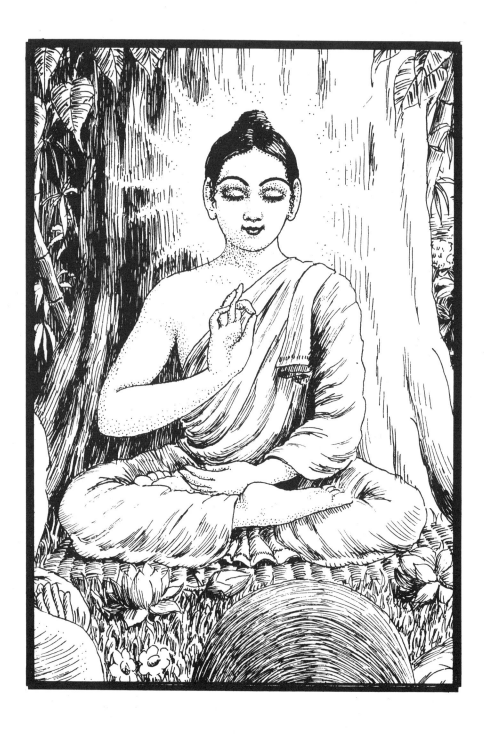

BUDDHISM

*"The eating of meat extinguishes the seed
of great compassion."*

—Mahaparinirvana Sutra

Buddhism, as practiced today, is a system of doctrine and technique developed by the followers of Siddhartha Gautama (563-483 B.C.), better known as "the Buddha." The title "Buddha" comes from the Sanskrit root *budh*, which means "to know," "to realize," or "to awaken." Thus, Buddha has come to mean "the enlightened one."

Practicing Buddhists today take various positions regarding what the Buddha taught; like Jesus, he committed nothing to writing. Yet his words were remembered by disciples and passed on to others. While many aspects of his teaching are still heavily debated within the community of Buddhists, two points are unanimously accepted: that he himself attained supreme enlightenment and that his compassion extended to everything that lives.

The late D. T. Suzuki, eminent authority on Buddhist teaching, comments in his *Essence of Buddhism*: "There are two pillars supporting the great edifice of Buddhism: *maha-prajna* ("great wisdom"), and *maha-karuna* ("great compassion"). The wisdom flows from the compassion and the compassion from the wisdom, for the two are one."[1] It is this, perhaps, that Dr. Suzuki had in mind when he wrote in his booklet *The Chain of Compassion*: "Buddhists must strive to teach respect and compassion for all creation—compassion is the foundation of their religion..."[2] In his own life, Buddha personified this great compassion, and the vegetarian way of life played an essential role in the wisdom he taught.

Enlightenment

According to Buddhist texts, Siddhartha Gautama, not yet known as Buddha, was the son of a great king who kept him isolated and protected from the iniquities of the outside world. In fact, as a youth Siddhartha led a charmed life within the high walls of his father's palace, oblivious to the miseries of material existence.

At the age of twenty-nine, however, Siddhartha ventured outside the palace confines and observed for the first time an old man, a diseased person, a dead body, and at last a *sannyasi* (a monk in the renounced order of life), who explained that Siddhartha's first three encounters were not rare scenes but rather the inevitable sorrows of all living beings in this world. Siddhartha grew sad and anxious and fell into deep contemplation. He resolved to discover a way by which people could conquer sorrow.

At first, he experimented with a life of fasting and severe penance. This made him so ill from lack of nourishment that he almost died. Self-affliction, he concluded, did not lead to the perfection he sought. In desperation, he became a wandering mendicant.

According to Buddhist tradition, one evening (probably around 531 B.C.), while meditating in the forest at Buddh Gaya, Siddhartha is said to have achieved a preliminary stage of enlightenment. That is, he was able to see utterly that material existence was illusory and that everything in this world was impermanent. It was also at Buddh Gaya, under the famous Bodhi Tree, that Siddhartha vowed to attain total enlightenment.

After practicing *sadhana* (spiritual disciplines) for six years, he reached his goal and composed his Four Noble Truths of material existence: suffering is universal in this world of change; suffering comes from desire; the extinction of desire brings about the extinction of suffering; the way to extinguish desire is to follow the Eight-fold Path. This path consists of right understanding, right purpose, right speech, right conduct, right work, right effort, right mindfulness and right contemplation. It is also known as the Middle Path (between excessive attachment and excessive renunciation of the world) and was meant to bring one beyond the realm of suffering and into *shunyata*, or "the void." The Buddha's philosophy, then, was one that espoused the cessation of suffering for all beings—and this naturally included, especially in early Buddhism, the suffering of animals.

The above is a simplification of Buddha's teaching; it is, however, all that is known for certain about his method of attaining enlightenment. There is one other teaching, too, that is considered fundamental to authentic Buddhist doctrine, and this is today still considered the First Precept of Buddhism: "Do not kill, but rather preserve and cherish all life."

Respect for All Things That Live

There is an ancient poem, reputed to be the only text ever written by Buddha himself:

> Creatures without feet have my love. And likewise those who have two feet; and those, too, who have many feet. Let creatures all, all things that live, all beings of whatever kind, see nothing that will bode them ill. May naught of evil come to them.

It is interesting to note that in the same century that Buddha taught this doctrine of contemplation and nonviolence, similar ideas were being taught in China by Confucius, in Persia by Zoroaster, in Greece by Pythagoras, in Jerusalem by Isaiah, and elsewhere in India by Mahavira.

While Buddhism flourished in the south of India, Jainism, as preached by Mahavira, flourished in the north. The Jains were so strict about the doctrine of noninjury that they would carefully examine anything they ate to avoid accidentally swallowing worms or insects—not for their own health but for the sake of the creatures. Both Jain and Buddhist monks carried strainers with their begging bowls to strain their water, lest they inadvertently swallow some small creature while drinking.

Although the Jains are traditionally stricter than the Buddhists in regard to noninjury and *ahimsa* principles, one should be aware just how this leniency in Buddhist tradition evolved. After Buddha's physical demise, early followers and scribes decided that his teachings actually emphasized "intent" over "action." The practical implications of this were far-reaching. According to their interpretation, an aspiring Buddhist could, for example, eat meat, provided the killing had been done by someone else. Notwithstanding, Buddha himself clearly discouraged meat-eating—his earliest biographers say that he looked upon the desire to eat meat as an "ignorant craving" (*trishna*).[3]

Buddha demanded his followers not eat meat under the following three conditions: if the follower personally saw the animal being killed; if he consented to its slaughter; or if he knew it was specifically being killed for him. This is the generally accepted view of Buddha's attitude toward meat-eating in all major Buddhist denominations.

While some branches of the Buddhist community today believe that dietary standards need not be so strict, others adamantly maintain that to eat the flesh of animals is certainly violent and thus non-Buddhist. Throughout history, this latter point of view has been held by many of the greatest exponents of Buddhist thought, such as Ashoka (268-223 B.C.) and Harsha (fl. fifth century A.D.), both strongly committed vegetarians and powerful political leaders. Emperor Ashoka, in fact, declared in one of his famous Pillar Edicts, "I have enforced the law against killing certain animals....The greatest progress of righteousness among men comes from the exhortation in favor of non-injury to life and abstention from killing living beings."[4]

The Buddhist view of animals is perhaps best illustrated in the Jataka stories, which tell of Buddha's previous incarnations in animal as well as human forms. Buddha himself is said to be the original narrator of these stories, which stress that not just Buddha but all people have been in animal form at one time or another. The stories teach that all creatures thus have the capacity for enlightenment in some future birth, and that killing an animal is therefore as heinous as killing a human being.

With the popularization and growth of the Buddhist community, a more permissive interpretation of *ahimsa* arose, overshadowing Buddha's original teaching of the underlying spiritual unity of all creation. It was at this point that "intent" superseded "action," and meat-eating became acceptable among Buddhists.

"Was the animal specifically killed for me?" the practicing Buddhist might ask. "If not," he reasoned, "then I may certainly partake of its flesh."

There is some truth to the predominance of "intent" over "action" in early Buddhist teaching.[5] However, that same school also insists that the practicing Buddhist have nothing to do with the destruction of life in any manner. This is especially so in Mahayana texts, as we shall soon see. Thus, while a monk, for instance, may not consciously be killing an animal when he accepts meat (as he begs alms from the householder), he is, in a very real sense, supporting the killing by accepting the flesh. He does not, in any case, discourage the meat-eating, and the worldly householder, who is dependent on him for proper knowledge, remains uninformed. The monk never tells him of his duty to avoid the killing of animals. By his complacency, by his emphasis of "intent" over "action," even the monk has become implicated in the killing.

A further explanation for the widespread acceptance of meat-eating by Buddhists is its apparent consistency with the Middle Path, which espouses a balance between renunciation and sensual pleasure. If one is eating meat, one is not practicing the intense austerity of fasting, and one is not necessarily gorging oneself either.

Still, it should be noted that Mahayana, perhaps the most important and widely practiced form of Buddhism today, boasts many texts inculcating the vegetarian ideal. Some of the Mahayanic works are said to contain direct quotes from Buddha. The *Lankavatara,* the *Surangama,* and the *Brahmajala,* to name a few, all support vegetarianism. Here is one example from the *Lankavatara:*

> For the sake of love of purity, the *bodhisattva* ("enlightened soul") should refrain from eating flesh, which is born from semen, blood, etc. For fear of causing terror to living beings let the *bodhisattva,* who is disciplining himself to attain compassion, refrain from eating flesh....It is not true that meat is proper food and permissible when the animal was not killed by himself, when he did not order others to kill it, when it was not specifically meant for him....Again, there may be some people in the future who...being under the influence of the taste for meat will string together in various ways many sophisticated arguments to defend meat-eating....But...meat-eating in any form, in any manner, and in any place is unconditionally and once and for all prohibited...Meat-eating I have not permitted to anyone, I do not permit, I will not permit.[6]

Further, the *Surangama Sutra* states:

> The reason for practicing *dhyana* ("meditation") and seeking to attain *samadhi* ("mystic perfection") is to escape from the suffering of life. But in seeking to escape from suffering ourselves, why should we inflict it upon others? Unless you can so control your minds that even the thought of brutal unkindness and killing is abhorrent, you will never be able to escape from the bondage of the world's life...After my *parinirvana* ("supreme enlightenment") in the final *kalpa* ("era") different kinds of ghosts will be encountered everywhere deceiving people and teaching them that they can eat meat and still attain enlighenment....How can a *bhikshu* ("seeker"), who hopes to become a deliverer of others, himself be living on the flesh of other sentient beings?[7]

Buddha in the Vedic Scriptures

It is significant that 2,500 years before Buddha was born, his life and mission were predicted in the *Bhagavata Purana,* or *Shrimad Bhagavatam.* Written by Vyasadeva, compiler of the Vedas and author of their classic commentary, *Vedanta Sutra,* the *Shrimad Bhagavatam* contains the essence of all Vedic knowledge and foretells the appearance of God's incarnations; the *Bhagavatam* lists them all—past, present, and future incarnations—along with distinguishing traits and a summary of their purpose in this world. Concerning Buddha, the 5,000-year-old *Bhagavatam* states:

tatah kalau sampravritte
sammohaya sura-dvisham
buddho namnanjana-sutah
kikateshu bhavishyati

In the beginning of the age of Kali, the Personality of Godhead will appear in the province of Gaya as Lord Buddha, the son of Anjana, to bewilder the demons who are always envious of the devotees of the Lord. (S.B. 1.3.24)

By textual reference, therefore, Buddha may properly be considered an incarnation (*avatara*) of the Supreme Godhead. Further, the word *bhavishyati,* "will appear," is especially significant, for it indicates that the event was to take place in the future. Buddha did indeed appear as the son of Anjana in the province of Gaya, some 2,500 years later.

A delineation of Buddha's mission appears in the works of Jayadeva Goswami, a renowned spiritual master and poet of the late twelfth century. In his popular devotional song *Gita Govinda,* in praise of ten prominent incarnations of God, Jayadeva wrote:

nindasi yajna-vidher ahaha sruti-jatam
sadaya-hridaya darsita-pasu-ghatam
keshava-dhrita-buddha-sarira
jaya jagadisha hare

Oh my Lord! Oh Personality of Godhead! All glories unto You! You compassionately appeared in the form of Lord Buddha to condemn the animal sacrifices recommended in the Vedic literature.

At the time of Buddha's manifestation in this world, the practice of Vedic religion had become somewhat debased. The people of India had deviated from the central purpose of the Vedas, which was devotion to the Supreme Being, and were indulging in mass slaughter of animals under the pretext of Vedic sacrifice. The esoteric meaning of such sacrifice is handed down in disciplic succession (*parampara*), and unless one is taught by a pure representative of such a disciplic line, his understanding of Vedic knowledge will be incomplete and imperfect.

Such was the case at the time of Buddha, and the wanton slaughter of animals—along with the eating of their flesh—became the religious doctrine of the ill-informed Vedic followers. Buddha's injunctions stopped this wholesale slaughter of animals, and authentic Indian Buddhism is still remembered for its emphasis on nonviolence and reverence for all life.

The Death of Buddha

As Buddhism spread to many lands, so did many misconceptions regarding Buddhism and vegetarianism. The events surrounding the death of Buddha are a good example. There is a Buddhist tradition, for instance, declaring that Buddha died from eating a piece of rancid meat. Such traditions ignore the many strong Buddhist texts advocating vegetarianism. Nineteenth-century scholarship has revealed that it was not meat but a poisonous truffle (a type of mushroom) that caused the death of the Enlightened One. There is considerable evidence to support this. The original Pali word, which is often mistranslated as "meat," or more specifically, "pig's flesh," is *sukara-maddava*. However, scholarly research has long since revealed that the Pali word for "pig's flesh" would be *sukara-mamsa*, and that the word used in connection with Buddha's death, *sukara-maddava*, actually refers to "a pig's delight."[8] Truffles, or a local delicacy known as "pignuts," are now generally accepted as the food Buddha ate at his last meal.

Nineteenth-century Buddhist expert Carolina A. Davids, wife of the well-known scholar Rhys C. Davids, offers a cogent argument in her definitive work, *A Manual of Buddhism:* "A food compound of pig-flesh (*sukaramamsa*) does occur once in the scriptures, in a *sutta* [verse] of a curiously unworthy kind, where a householder, in inviting Gotama to dine, goes through quite a menu in refrained detail! *Maddava* is nowhere else associated with meat. ...We have here a dish...of a root, such as truffles, much sought by swine, and which may have been called 'pig's joy.' Such a root we actually have—this the critics did not know—in our 'pignut,'... the little nut-shaped bulbous roots of which, called also 'earthnuts,' are liked by both pigs and children."[9]

Most Buddhist scholars today, both vegetarian and non-vegetartian, lean toward this perspective and tend to admit that the theory of Buddha's eating "pig flesh" as his last food was a careless assumption, with absolutely no scholarly substantiation.

Buddhism in China and Japan

According to *The Encyclopedia of Buddhism*, "In China and Japan the eating of meat was looked upon as an evil and was ostracized....The eating of meat gradually ceased [c. fifth century A.D.] and this tended to become general. It became a matter of course not to use any kind of meat in the meals of temples and monasteries."[10] In fact, monks who ate even fish were disparagingly referred to as *namagusubozu*—"an unholy monk smelling of raw fish!"[11]

When Buddhism spread to China during the Han dynasty (206 B.C.-A.D. 220), Confucianism and Taoism were already established. The Chinese of this period primarily worshiped the ancestral family, paying homage according to strict dietary rules and an intricate array of religious doctrines. Certain foods, for example, including pork, which made the breath "obnoxious to the ancestors,"[12] were frowned upon. In other words, some vegetarian or quasi-vegetarian codes already existed in China.

Buddhism was soon introduced into Japan, where in the sixth century it began to gain a stronghold. This was an exceptionally propitious time for such an event; the Japanese court had by then incorporated much of China's culture. Classical Chinese was adopted as the literary language, and China's traditional religions—including Buddhism—were embraced.

The indigenous religion of Japan, Shinto, was a faith as old as Japan itself, essentially pantheistic in its worship of nature. The Buddhism of China fit nicely into the Shinto scheme of things, and a kind of merger between Shinto and Chinese Buddhism has endured in Japan to this day. In fact, the Buddhism with which most people are today familiar is based more or less on this merger, as opposed to the original form of Buddhism indigenous to India. However it is this original form that accentuates vegetarianism and kindness to all creatures.

Significant traces of vegetarian thinking, however, are found throughout Shinto as well. The source of all creation and the essence of the universe, for instance, is called *kami,* according to Shinto doctrine, and to attain realization of this supreme reality, both spiritual and material purification are essential. The body must be purged of contaminated elements and only *sattvik,* pure foods (mainly vegetarian), may be consumed. Today, during thanksgiving festivals at Shinto shrines, special offerings are made, including rice, rice cakes, sake, vegetables, fish and birds. In the early days of Shinto, however, no animal food was offered because of the taboo against shedding blood in the sacred area of the shrine.[13] Here again we discover evidence of a religion's original intent to avoid the killing and eating of animal flesh. As in most other religions, too, we see here that later interpretations of Shinto eventually relaxed the mandate for mercy and compassion.

While the eating of meat—especially fish—is now commonplace in Japan, the deeply religious still consider meat-eating a lower activity, and meat-eaters are still sometimes known as outcasts. For example, no meat or fish is ever eaten in a Zen Buddhist monastery, where Zen masters retain their reputation for strict self-discipline and their steady adherence to ancient laws.

Contemporary Buddhist movements, such as the Buddhists Concerned for Animal Rights, are also interested in reestablishing vegetarian principles in the Buddhist tradition. And such Buddhist denominations as the Cao Dai sect, which originated in South Vietnam, now boasts some two million followers, all of whom are vegetarian.

If we study Buddhism as it was originally practiced in India, and if we are aware of the circumstances surrounding its adaptation in China and Japan, what emerges is this: original forms of Buddhism taught compassion for all life and aversion to cruelty in any form. Like other Eastern traditions, it unambiguously exhorted its followers to accept vegetarianism as essential to personal spiritual awakening. We have also seen that concessions to meat-eating in the Buddhist tradition are attributable to the rationalization of "intent" over "action," and to the problems incurred by the transferal of a religious culture to a new land. Consistently, however, *ahimsa,* or reverence for all life, has stood as a central pillar supporting the houses of Eastern religious thought, particularly Buddhism.

REFERENCES

1. D. T. Suzuki, *The Essence of Buddhism,* 2nd edition (London, The Buddhist Society, 1947), pp. 34-35.

2. D. T. Suzuki, *The Chain of Compassion* (Cambridge, Mass., Cambridge Buddhist Association, 1966), p. 13.

3. Dudley Giehl, *Vegetarianism: A Way of Life* (New York, Harper and Row, 1979), p. 172.

4. "The Seventh Pillar Edict" in *Sources of Indian Tradition,* trans. William de Barry et al. (New York, Columbia University Press, 1958).

5. Unto Tahtinen, *op. cit.,* p. 107.

6. *The Lankavatara Sutra,* trans. D. T. Suzuki (London, Routledge, 1932).

7. *A Buddhist Bible,* ed. Dwight Goddard (New York, Dutton, 1952), pp. 264-265.

8. Philip Kapleau, *To Cherish All Life: A Buddhist Case for Becoming Vegetarian* (New York, Harper & Row, 1982), p. 24.

9. Carolina A. Davids, *A Manual of Buddhism* (London, Sheldon, 1932), p. 260.

10. Philip Kapleau, *op. cit.,* p. 34.

11. *Ibid.*

12. John Cook, *Diet and Your Religion* (New York, Woodbridge Press, 1976), p. 35.

13. *Ibid.,* p. 41.

HINDUISM

Chapter 7

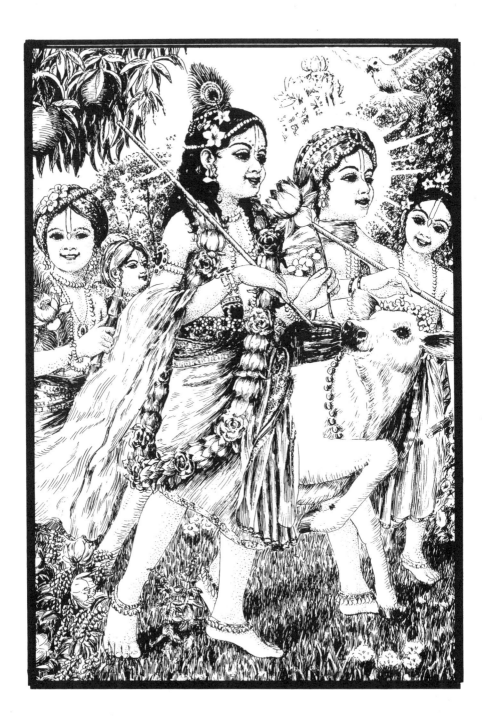

HINDUISM

"Having well considered the origin of flesh-foods,
and the cruelty
of fettering and slaying corporeal beings,
let man entirely abstain
from eating flesh."

—Manusmriti 5.49

Asia is the continent of superlatives: it has the largest land area, the highest mountains, the greatest number of people, the first civilization, the first writing, the earliest agriculture, the first cities, the first codified legal system, the oldest continuous monarchy, and the oldest religions in the world. Hinduism, the oldest of all Asian religions, is also the earliest and strongest propounder of vegetarianism.

While other major world religions are traceable to one particular founder, Hinduism has its beginnings in such remote antiquity that it cannot be traced to any one individual. Its roots, however, are firmly planted in the ancient Vedic texts. The word "Hindu" is not actually found anywhere in the Vedic scriptures. The term was introduced by Muslims from neighboring Afghanistan, Baluchistan and Persia and referred to people living across the River Sindhu, which borders India's northwest provinces. These Muslim tribes pronounced their "s's" like "h's," and thus "Sindhus" became "Hindus." The river has since been renamed the Indus.

The term "Hindu" is vague, and even a misnomer, for it refers to people who settled near the River Sindhu, a people who actually held a vast array of religious beliefs. There is no one "Hindu religion." And the

91

original Vedic system is actually quite different from contemporary Hinduism. Both the old and the new, however, converge harmoniously in regard to vegetarianism. The following are but a few of the thousands of Vedic injunctions against meat-eating:

> One who partakes of human flesh, the flesh of a horse or of another animal, and deprives others of milk by slaughtering cows, O King, if such a fiend does not desist by other means, then you should not hesitate to cut off his head. (Rig Veda, 10.87.16)

> You must not use your God-given body for killing God's creatures, whether they are human, animal or whatever. (Yajur Veda, 12.32)

> One should be considered dear, even by the animal kingdom. (Atharva Veda, 17.1.4)

> Those noble souls who practice meditation and other yogic ways, who are ever careful about all beings, who protect all animals, are the ones who are actually serious about spiritual practices. (Atharva Veda, 19.48.5)

> By not killing any living being, one becomes fit for salvation. (Manusmriti, 6.60)

> The purchaser of flesh performs *himsa* [violence] by his wealth; he who eats flesh does so by enjoying its taste; the killer does *himsa* by actually tying and killing the animal. Thus, there are three forms of killing. He who brings flesh or sends for it, he who cuts off the limbs of an animal, and he who purchases, sells, or cooks flesh and eats it—all of these are to be considered meat-eaters. (Mahabharata, Anu. 115:40)

> He who desires to augment his own flesh by eating the flesh of other creatures lives in misery in whatever species he may take his birth. (Mahabharata, Anu. 115:47)

> Those who are ignorant of real dharma and, though wicked and haughty, account themselves virtuous, kill animals without any feeling of remorse or fear of punishment. Further, in their next lives, such sinful persons will be eaten by the same creatures they have killed in this world. (Shrimad Bhagavatam, 11.5.14)

Animal Sacrifices

Although verses such as the above clearly advocate vegetarianism, there was another current in the Vedic tradition that permitted animal sacrifice under special circumstances. (Buddha, it may be remembered, condemned such animal sacrifices in his reform of Hinduism.) These sacrifices were intended to attract meat-eaters to a more holy way of life by getting them to follow scriptural rules and regulations. Unlike other world scriptures that temporized in regard to meat-eating, however, the Vedic literature emphasizes that this is an inferior mode of worship.

In certain parts of the Vedic literature there are descriptions of rituals and ceremonies in which a horse is offered to God in a sacrificial arena. The purpose of these rituals was not to sanctify the eating of horse flesh. Rather, it was to prove the efficacy of Vedic mantra (mystical sound vibration).

An old horse would be led into a fire of sacrifice, qualified *brahmanas* (priests) would chant the sacred mantra, and the horse would then emerge in a rejuvenated body. The animal was never harmed, only rejuvenated. Today, of course, there are no qualified priests to perform such a complicated, mystical sacrifice, and the Vedas themselves specify that these rituals were only for an earlier age.

Another type of animal sacrifice mentioned in the Vedas involved a goat, which was to be killed in the presence of the goddess Kali. This procedure is described in the *Markandeya Purana*, a scripture that prescribes rituals for the gradual elevation of the spiritually ignorant. Those who were more spiritually evolved would offer red flowers to the goddess instead of a blood sacrifice, and in this way appease her with the facsimile of color.[1]

It is interesting, too, that these texts describing goat sacrifice only sanctioned the eating of flesh offered on the altar. Much like early Judaism, which originally only granted the eating of meat offered sacrificially at the first Temple, the Vedic and Puranic literature never endorsed the wholesale slaughter of animals so prevalent today.

Worshippers of Kali were obliged to chant the Sanskrit word for meat (*mamsa*) into the goat's ear before slitting its throat. The word carries deep meaning. Etymologically, *mamsa* is broken down into *mam* ("me") and *sa* ("he"). According to traditional Indian philology, the implication is as follows: "As I eat him now, so he will eat me in the future."[2] This is an example of the law of karma: for every action, there is an equal and opposite reaction. While the word karma literally means "act," it also implies causality (see Afterword).

The complete Sanskrit verse in which *mamsa* originally appears is as follows:

> *mamsa sa bhakshayitamutra*
> *yasya mamsam ihadmy aham*
> *etan mamsaya mamsatvam*
> *pravadanti manisinaha*

That creature whose flesh I am eating here and now will consume me in the next life. Thus, meat is called *mamsa,* as described by learned authorities.

The Sanskrit noun *pashu-ghna* ("he who kills the body"), a word that is also intimately connected to meat-eating and allied concepts, can apply to both "meat-eater" and "one who commits suicide." This reinforces the notion that a severe reaction awaits anyone who eats meat.

In his instructions to King Prachinabarhi, who was enamored by opulent animal sacrifices, the sage Narada Muni lays bare the karmic reaction to meat-eating: "O ruler of the citizens, my dear King, please see in the sky those animals which you have sacrificed, without compassion and without mercy, in the sacrificial arena. All these animals are awaiting your death so that they can avenge the injuries you have inflicted upon them. After you die, they will angrily pierce your body with iron horns and then eat your flesh." (*Shrimad Bhagavatam,* 4.25.7-8) This, again, is consistent with the traditional understanding of the word *mamsa.*

Despite popular knowledge of meat-eating's adverse effects, the non-vegetarian diet became increasingly widespread among Hindus after the two major invasions by foreign powers, first the Muslims and later the British. With them came the desire to be "civilized," to eat as did the *saheeb.* Those actually trained in Vedic knowledge, however, never adopted a meat-oriented diet, and the pious Hindu still observes vegetarian principles as a matter of religious duty. (Eighty-three percent of India's 680 million people are Hindu, the majority of whom are vegetarian.)[3]

The large number of Hindu vegetarians can be attributed, in great measure, to the very clear teaching of universal compassion found in the Vedic literature. Acknowledging two distinct levels of ethical consideration, the Vedas promote *sarva-bhuta-hita* ("devotion to the good of all creatures") over *loka-hita* ("devotion to the good of humanity"). The first ethical system, say the Vedas, includes the second. If one cares for all living creatures, then one naturally cares for humanity as well.

The Vedic viewpoint is that a person should see the same life-force in all living entities—regardless of "outer dress" (the body). Those who cannot understand the principle of life in lesser beings may then eventually misunderstand what the life-force is altogether and lose their sense of humanity. Accordingly, *sarva-bhuta-hita,* or the desire to do good for all creatures, is the superior code of ethics delineated in the Vedas and remains a central tenet of Hinduism.

Cow Protection

Of all creatures, the cow is given a special place in the Indian religious tradition. In the words of Mahatma Gandhi, "Mother cow is, in many ways, better than the mother who gave us birth. Our mother gives us milk for a couple of years, and expects us to serve her when we grow up. Mother cow expects nothing of us but grass and grain. Our mother often falls ill and expects service from us. Mother cow rarely falls ill. Our mother, when she dies, expects expenses of burial or cremation. Mother cow is useful dead as when alive."[4]

Traditionally, the cow is also considered dear to Lord Krishna, Who is glorified in Vedic and post-Vedic texts as the Supreme Lord. Vaishnavism, or the worship of Vishnu or Krishna, is the original religion of the Vedas, and Krishna's love for the cow is celebrated throughout the Vedic literature. It is no wonder, therefore, that we find great emphasis on *ahimsa* and especially cow protection in the earliest parts of the Vedic canon.

According to India's traditional scriptural histories, the original cow, Mother Surabhi, was one of the treasures churned from the cosmic ocean, and "the five products of the cow" (*pancha-gavya*)— milk, curd, ghee, urine and dung—were all considered purifying.[5] Despite the veneration bestowed upon her, there is no "cow-goddess" in the Hindu religion, as is generally supposed, and no temples are ever constructed in the cows' honor. Rather, the cow is respected in her own right as one of the seven mothers,[6] because she offers her milk as does one's natural mother.

The cow plays a central role in the Vedic ideal for humanity: "simple living and high thinking," a life close to nature and God. And until fairly recently in India's history, most of the people lived on tracts of land suitable for complete self-sufficiency. Cows thus played—and continue to play—a central role in India's economy. For example, cow dung serves as an inexpensive fertilizer. Stored in underground tanks, it also generates methane gas that is used for heating and cooking. Cow dung is also an effective disinfectant and is used both as a poultice and a cleansing agent.

For these and other reasons, the Vedic lexicon *Nighantu* offers nine names for the cow, three of which—*aghnya* ("not to be killed"), *ahi* ("not to be killed") and *aditi* ("not to be cut")—specifically forbid slaughter. These synonyms for "cow" are found throughout the Vedic literature and are summarized in the epic work *Mahabharata:* "The very name of the cows is *aghnya*, indicating that they should never be slaughtered. Who, then, could slay them? Surely, one who kills a cow or a bull commits the most heinous crime." (*Shantiparva* 262.47)

Vegetarianism and Nonviolence

That vegetarianism has always been widespread in India is clear from the earliest Vedic texts. This was observed by the ancient traveler Megasthenes and also by Fa-hsien, a Chinese Buddhist monk who, in the fifth century, traveled to India in order to obtain authentic copies of the scriptures.

These scriptures unambiguously support the meatless way of life. In the *Mahabharata,* for instance, the great warrior Bhishma explains to Yudhisthira, eldest of the Pandava princes, that the meat of animals is like the flesh of one's own son, and that the foolish person who eats meat must be considered the vilest of human beings.[7] The *Mahabharata* emphasizes this point. The eating of "dirty" food, it warns, is not as terrible as the eating of flesh[8] (it must be remembered that the *brahmanas* of ancient India exalted cleanliness to a divine principle).

Similarly, the *Manusmriti* declares that one should "refrain from eating all kinds of meat," for such eating involves killing and leads to karmic bondage (*bandha*).[9]

Elsewhere in the Vedic literature, the last of the great Vedic kings, Maharaja Pariksit, is quoted as saying that "only the animal-killer cannot relish the message of the Absolute Truth."[10] Therefore, the Vedas inform us, to obtain spiritual knowledge, one must begin with being vegetarian.

The *Mahabharata,* cited above, is often associated with another epic work, the *Ramayana.* Together, these two texts are considered the greatest literary works of the East, each strong in its support of vegetarianism. The *Ramayana* informs us that elevated souls, such as descendants of the demigod Ikshvaku, shun meat-eating and violence in any form (*ahimsa-rati*).[11] Of course, the Ikshvaku dynasty, and other great dynasties of India, were not impractical: when necessary, they would employ *kshatriya* (military) methods to defend their kingdom. But it should be noted that the true *kshatriya* was never violent in an antagonistic sense. Rather, he "protected others from violence," as the etymology of the word implies (from the root *kshat,* which means "hurt," and *trayate,* "to give protection.").[12]

Indeed, the *Bhagavad Gita* teaches that one should not be fanatical about nonviolence and that total nonviolence is in fact an impossibility. Material nature forces us to commit violence, for even breathing necessitates the killing of countless microorganisms. "Nonviolence in politics may be a diplomacy," the *Gita* teaches, "but it is never a factor or principle."[13]

Mahatma Gandhi also acknowledged that nonviolence may exist within violence—albeit in very rare exceptions. "I have come to see," wrote Gandhi, "what I did not so clearly before, that there is nonviolence in violence....I had not fully realized the duty of restraining a drunkard from doing evil, of killing a dog in agony or one infected with rabies. In all these instances, violence is in fact nonviolence."[14]

Nonviolence, in the Vedic tradition, has to be practiced with common sense, guided by scriptures and qualified teachers. Discussing the implications of the *Gita*'s teachings in this regard, Indian historian S. Dasgupta asks: if a dangerous beast enters a cattle shed, should one kill the beast or allow it to destroy the valuable cattle? Kill the beast, he concludes, for the principal objective is to maintain social order and the well-being of the people.[15] Higher forms of nonviolence may include being "violent" for a greater good. This is the *kshatriya* principle. According to the *Gita,* this principle supercedes any abstraction, such as unqualified nonviolence that may result in more harm done than good.

The fundamental principle of all Vedic injunctions, however, is that everything must be done in pursuit of God's will. For example, even the action of hunting (*mrigaya*), which is considered sinful, can be counteracted by austerity (*tapas*) and surrender to God (*mad-upashraya*).[16] This surrender is the crucial point in Vedic religion. To give some indication of its importance, the *Varaha Purana* relates a story in which an ignorant but sincere hunter kills only one animal a day and offers part of the flesh to God, for it is his misguided belief that his offering purifies the killing. In the story there is also a vegetarian forest dweller, a farmer who harvests grain. The Vedas recognize grain as a lower yet conscious life form, and in the process of accumulating grain, the farmer kills more living beings (in the form of seeds and plants) than the hunter. The farmer, however, never offers anything to God. The story concludes that he was therefore more sinful than the hunter and guilty of *maha-himsa,* the highest violence, for he is one "who eats flesh without ritual offering." This story, the Purana tells us, is not to endorse meat-eating, which is sinful, but to eulogize offering food to God, which eradicates all sin.[17]

"The Lord's Mercy"

According to the Vedic scriptures, one should offer all foods as a sacrifice to God: "...all that you do, all that you eat, all that you offer and give away, as well as all austerities that you may perform, should be done as an offering unto Me." (*Bhagavad Gita* 9.27)

One should not conclude from this, however, that everything is offerable (as our simple hunter wrongly believed). The *Gita* specifies exactly what should be offered: "If one offers Me with love and devotion a leaf, a flower, fruit or water, I will accept it." (B.G. 9.26) There are other references in the Vedas confirming that fruits, vegetables, grain, nuts and dairy products are fit for human consumption. Followers of the *Gita* refrain from offering meat, fish, poultry or eggs, for these are not sanctioned by either the scriptures or the Vedic prophets. According to the Vedic tradition, then, submission to God's word and the words of His prophets and sages invariably leads to vegetarianism.

The *Bhagavad Gita* further declares that one who lovingly offers his food to God, according to scriptural guidelines, is freed from all sinful reactions and consequent rebirth in the material world: "The devotees of the Lord are released from all kinds of sins because they eat food which is offered first in sacrifice. Others, who prepare food for personal sense enjoyment, verily eat only sin." (B.G. 3.13)

The remnants of such devotional offerings are called *prasadam* (literally, "The Lord's Mercy"). In India, the largest temples, such as Shri Rangam in South India and Jagannath Mandir, the main temple in Puri (state of Orissa), all freely distribute sanctified vegetarian foods (*prasadam*) for the benefit of the multitudes who approach the holy shrines daily. One of the most celebrated Vedic sages, Narada Muni, was inspired to embark on the spiritual path by tasting delicious vegetarian foods offered to the Lord.

Of the many contemporary movements based on Vedic philosophy and religion, followers of the International Society for Krishna Consciousness (ISKCON) are noteworthy for the support of vegetarianism. In the many ISKCON temples and restaurants, only *prasadam*, sanctified vegetarian food, is served to the guests.

Animals and Spirituality

Long before St. Francis was declared the patron saint of animals, the sages of ancient India had already recognized spirituality in all living species. Vedic texts even describe incarnations of God in various nonhuman forms, after which each of the many species of life on our planet is modeled. Some of the most popular incarnations represented in India are the boar, the tortoise, the fish, and the horse—there is even a half man/half lion incarnation. (Vedic literature does not promote polytheism; rather, the Vedas affirm that it is the same one God who appears in various forms.)

Further, the Vedic viewpoint fully acknowledges—albeit in specific circumstances—the ability of ordinary animals to achieve exalted states of spirituality. This is attributable to the fact that the Vedic vision of spirituality is not limited to the human form. Followers of the Vedas identify neither themselves nor any other living creature with the external body. Rather, they see the same eternal soul within each bodily shell, imbued with the same spiritual perfection.

The hypocrisy of claiming to be religious while adhering to a vision other than the one described above was brought out by Steven J. Gelberg in a thought-provoking paper delivered to the Assembly of the World's Religions I: "Because he cannot really sense his own soul, the mundane religionist cannot sense it in other creatures and so thinks nothing of feasting on their slaughtered remains. Insisting that some living creatures have life but no soul, he inadvertently assumes the ideologic posture of the materialist, who reduces life to a mere biologic function. Under the sway of this contradiction, he fondles one lesser creature and slaughters another, pampering one as his pet and cannibalizing the other as his dinner. Devoid of even rudimentary consciousness of spirit, he remains blissfully unaware of his sin.

"Belief in souls in animals aside," Gelberg continues, "the mundane religionist lacks the moral keenness and simple compassion to be sickened by the bloody cruelty which he tacitly endorses as a human carnivore. Due to dullness, he remains unaware that the creature he blithely eats had to endure unspeakable suffering in the slaughterhouse—suffering for which he himself, as its chief beneficiary, is responsible. His scriptures enjoin 'Thou Shalt Not Kill,' but he kills with blind, grinding routine. 'As you did it to one of the least of these my brethren,' says Jesus, 'you did it to Me.'"[18]

Gelberg's point is clear: the difference between religion with a small "r" and Religion with a capital "R" is how successfully it encompasses all living beings.

The Vedas say that the living soul transmigrates, from body to body, from species to species, until it finally reaches the human form, equipped with reason and the ability to inquire into Absolute Truth. Exercising that human prerogative, one can end the cycle of repeated birth and death and attain the kingdom of God.

There are instances in India's Sanskrit scriptures where even souls in animal form achieved liberation from repeated incarnations. Here is an indication of how equitably animals are viewed in the Vedic texts, for this is the only world religion to declare that animals can reach the same supreme destination sought by humans.

These cases of "animal liberation" occur when the particular animal achieves the association of a great saint or an incarnation of God, and such instances testify to the importance of such holy association. The most recent examples in religious history occurred during the life of Shri Chaitanya Mahaprabhu, revered as an incarnation of Krishna Himself.[19] On pilgrimage in South India, Shri Chaitanya passed through the Jarikhanda Forest. The sixteenth-century Bengali text, *Shri Chaitanya Charitamrita*, describes that Chaitanya danced in love of God and chanted the holy names now popularly known as the Hare Krishna mantra: Hare Krishna, Hare Krishna, Krishna Krishna, Hare Hare, Hare Rama, Hare Rama, Rama Rama, Hare Hare. Seeing His ecstasy, the text relates, elephants, tigers, deer and birds chanted and danced with Him. Chaitanya's love of God overflowed, carrying the animals in its wake, and inspired the creatures of the forest to express their own love of God. They chanted in their own animal tongues and danced with Chaitanya all the while. Elephants roaring loudly and rocking their massive bodies back and forth mingled with the swaying of divinely intoxicated rhinoceros. And as the tigers and deer chanted and danced, the Vedic literature tells us, they embraced one another in ecstatic love, a scenario which can only be reminiscent of the Messianic prophecy in the biblical book of Isaiah: "...the wolf and the lamb shall feed together and the lion shall eat straw like the bullock. They shall not hurt nor destroy in all My holy mountain." (Isaiah 65:24-25)

Balabhadra Bhattacharya, Shri Chaitanya's servant, witnessed the whole spectacle and was struck with spiritual emotion. "These animals are not ordinary living entities," Balabhadra thought to himself. "They are special recipients of the Lord's mercy."[20]

While the previous narration reveals that animals can achieve a high level of spirituality in this world, the following story from the same text shows that animals can also attain the kingdom of God. The tale emphasizes Vaishnava compassion and the awareness that the soul is the same no matter what body it inhabits.

The story in the Bengali scripture begins by describing that Shri Chaitanya spent the latter portion of His life in Jagannath Puri, where His devotees from Bengal would make a yearly pilgrimage to visit Him. One devotee, Shivananda Sen, was in charge of seeing to the others' needs during the long and arduous journey, which, in those days, meant traveling by foot. One year, as Shivananda led the devotees out of Bengal, a dog tagged along.

"Here is a spirit-soul who wants to see Shri Chaitanya," he thought. "Let him come with us. What difference does it make that he is not born into the same species? He wants to see the Lord."

Shivananda took care of the dog throughout the long pilgrimage, personally feeding him prasadam every day. When it came time to travel a short distance by boat, Shivananda gladly consented to paying the additional fare for the dog, never thinking that it was unnecessary for the dog to see Shri Chaitanya.

To Shivananda's great dismay, the dog eventually ran away. But when at last the weary pilgrims reached Puri, they saw the dog sitting contentedly at Chaitanya's holy feet, and the master was feeding him coconut pulp from His own hand.

"Chant the name of Krishna!" Chaitanya told the dog, and the dog barked, "Krishna! Krishna!"

"This is very wonderful!" Shivananda said to the others. "This dog must be an eternal associate of the Lord. We were fortunate to have his association." The scripture relates that by Chaitanya's association the dog's love for God was reawakened, and that from his animal body he returned directly to the kingdom of God.[21] The *Shri Chaitanya Charitamrita* is today accepted as part of the Vedic canon by all believing Gaudiya Vaishnavas.

Here, then, is a religious tradition that emphasizes not only vegetarianism but also the spiritual equality of all living beings. If elephants can learn to dance with lions, and dogs can attain the kingdom of God, then their spiritual status is such that they should not be cruelly tortured or slaughtered. Vegetarianism is nothing less than the confirmation of this awareness that all living beings are spiritually equal.

REFERENCES

1. Lawrence A. Babb, *The Divine Hierarchy: Popular Hinduism in Central India* (New York, Columbia University Press, 1975), p. 225.

2. Explanation of *mamsa* appears in *Shrimad Bhagavatam* 11.5.14.

3. Julie Sahni, *Classic Indian Vegetarian and Grain Cooking* (New York, William Morrow and Company, Inc., 1985), p. 23.

4. Benjamin Walker, *The Hindu World* (New York, Praeger Publishers, 1968), p. 26.

5. A. L. Basham, *The Wonder That Was India* (New York, Grove Press, 1959), p. 319.

6. According to Vedic tradition, the seven mothers are one's natural mother, the midwife, the wife of the guru, the wife of the *brahmana*, the wife of the king, the earth and the cow.

7. *Mahabharata, Anusana-parva* 114.11.

8. *Mahabharata, Santi-parva* 141.88.

9. *Manusmriti* 5.49.

10. *Shrimad Bhagavatam* 10.1.4.

11. *Ramayana,* 5.31.4.

12. A. C. Bhaktivedanta Swami Prabhupada, *Bhagavad-Gita As It Is* (New York, Macmillan, 1972), pp. 113-114.

13. *Ibid.*

14. Quoted in Erik H. Erikson, *Gandhi's Truth* (New York, Norton, 1969), p. 374.

15. S. Dasgupta, *A History of Indian Philosophy,* Vol. II, (London, Cambridge University Press, 1932), pp. 508-509.

16. *Shrimad Bhagavatam,* 10.51.63.

17. *Varaha Purana,* 8.26-30.33.

18. Steven J. Gelberg, "The Transcendental Imperative: The Case for 'Otherworldly' Religion." Presented at "Assembly of the World's Religions 1: Recovering Our Classical Heritage." New Jersey, Nov. 15-21, 1985, pp. 7-8.

19. Shri Chaitanya Mahaprabhu, according to the Vedic scriptures and the Vaishnava tradition, is Krishna Himself in the role of His own devotee. Some 500 years ago He appeared in Bengal, India, to inaugurate the meditative process of chanting the holy name of the Lord.

20. A. C. Bhaktivedanta Swami Prabhupada, *Shri Chaitanya Charitamrita,* 17 Vols., (Los Angeles, Bhaktivedanta Book Trust, 1975), *Antya-lila,* Vol. 1, Chapter 1.

21. *Ibid., Madhya-lila,* Vol. 7, Chapter 1

AFTERWORD

Vegetarianism should be kept in perspective; it is one religious imperative among many. Although based on the primary spiritual principle of compassion and empathy for all creatures, it is not an end in itself. It is a *part* of the religious process, augmenting essential spiritual practices such as prayer, meditation, proper behavior toward fellow humans, and service to God.

Indeed, militant animal rights activists who cause harm to scientists engaged in vivisection or who destroy animal experimentation laboratories are guilty of crimes comparable to those of which they accuse meat-eaters and animal abusers. They readily cause harm and destruction while speaking of love and peace. They seek to save animals by wreaking havoc among humans. It is no wonder, therefore, that those who witness their activities consider them hypocritical and misled. Granted, such radical activists represent a minority among those who see the wisdom in having compassion for animals, and, among those who would engage in such violence, fewer still are those who do so for religious reasons. But even if there is one—it is one too many. A religious vegetarian should be a balanced person, one who has compassion and love for animals, but no less for humans.

Overview

This book has attempted to show that there is much in each of the world's major religions to endorse vegetarianism and the compassionate treatment of animals. Ignorance of this fact, especially in the Western

103

world, has kept our four-footed, feathered and scaly kin in our kitchens instead of our hearts. In America, for example, one who adheres to any of the current Judaeo-Christian faiths would be hard-pressed to make a case for animal rights as a plausible concern, worthy, perhaps, of serious consideration.

The mainstream seems quite comfortable with its meat-and-potatoes spirituality. Nonetheless, prominent voices from within the religious community are beginning to speak on behalf of the creatures, making a convincing case for at least considering their plight. Richard Schwartz's excellent book *Judaism and Vegetarianism* and Andrew Linzey's *Christianity and the Rights of Animals* were ground-breakers, showing that scripture and tradition are quite supportive of the animal rights concern from within the Western religious milieu.

Why, then, do Western religious traditions seem, on the whole, to denounce animal rights and all that it stands for? One reason, perhaps, is the extreme view of some animal rights activists, as we've noted. But Schwartz and Linzey point to more fundamental problems, showing how the scriptures have been adjusted, maligned, interpolated, and interpreted to suit the whims of political and religious figures across the centuries. Some of these ideas have been addressed in this short work, but there is much literature dedicated to documenting these subjects in detail, and we have provided a bibliography for those interested in further research.

The Eastern religious traditions are more forthcoming in relation to animal rights. The Orient has, in general, managed to maintain at least a healthy reverence for all of God's creation, often extending this reverence to the point of vegetarianism. Because the Eastern religions are ancient—especially as represented in early Sanskrit and Pali texts—many scholars have been led to research Eastern scriptures with a view to finding the source of the animal rights sensibility. Since the five major world religions—Judaism, Christianity, Islam, Buddhism, and Hinduism—all originate in the East, academicians have especially considered Hinduism, the oldest of all Asian religions, to be an important starting place for their investigation of the spiritual origin of animal rights.

The principle of ethics found in the earliest Indian scriptures (the Vedas) is known, in ancient Sanskrit, as *sarva-bhuta-hita*, which means "kindness to all creatures," as opposed to the more limited vision of *loka-hita*, or "kindness to one's own species." The former ethical system, say the Vedas, includes the latter, and therefore it is to be embraced by those who are wise. Love of all creatures is a more inclusive ethic, and followers of the Vedic tradition were encouraged to develop this broad spiritual vision. Further, *ahimsa*, or "harmlessness," in all its forms, was to be adopted by progressive souls who wanted to develop spiritual acumen.

As Christopher Chapple notes in his book *Nonviolence to Animals, Earth, and Self in Asian Traditions,* modern scholarship has been surprisingly ineffectual when trying to discover the origins of *ahimsa.* Some scholars acknowledge an earlier Vedic origin, but most say it did not come into prominence until Buddhism; while still others say it can be attributed to the rise of Jainism. Two sources often cited are L. Alsdorf's *Beitrage zur Geschichte von Vegetarismus und Rinderverehrung in Indien* and Hanns-Peter Schmidt's *The Origin of Ahimsa.* These works emphasize social law as found in traditional Hindu law manuals. Although they mention the Jain proclivity for *ahimsa,* they are noncommittal about whether the concept originated with that religion. The authors also claim that Mahavira, the reputed founder of Jainism, was not a vegetarian, but this claim was convincingly refuted by Jain scholar H.R. Kapadia.

Schmidt assumes that the indigenous Indus Valley people could not have been vegetarian, since the bones of flesh animals were found in the ruins of Mohenjodaro and Harappa. He writes that "there are...no traces of similar ideas to be found among the non-Aryan population of India— not influenced by the Brahmanical culture—which could justify the assumption that *ahimsa* and vegetarianism did not originate from concep- tions evolved among the Aryans." His basic point is that since the remains of flesh animals in Mohenjodaro and Harappa seem to have been animals that were eaten, the local inhabitants were not vegetarian. Most modern scholars disagree with Schmidt. For example, Chapple notes that "...the presence of bones in a city's garbage does not mean that all its inhabitants ate meat. Within India to the present day, both carnivores and vegetarians coexist." Chapple's research into the *Mahabharata* (*Shanti Parvan*), wherein Bhishma and Yudhisthira discuss many theological subjects, including animal rights and vegetarianism, shows clearly the early Indian origins of *ahimsa* and its logical extension of the non-meat diet. Peter Schreiner has also examined the holy *Mahabharata* dialogue, and he comes to similar conclusions. It is the contention of this author, too, that the pri- mal origins of *ahimsa* can be found in India's ancient Vedic culture, which reached its culmination in her theistic traditions, such as Vaishnavism. Sincere adherents of all religions, if they drink deeply their own tradition, can find much with which to agree when Vaishnava sages proclaim, *ahimsa paro dharmo:* "Nonviolence is the highest religion."

Concluding Thoughts

Compassion for animals is an integral part of the Asian mindset and has been so throughout the annals of recorded history. Christopher Chapple elaborates: "The view of animals held by those in the Indian milieu differs radically from that held by those living in the European-Western technological matrix. Similar views are found in Hinduism, Buddhism, and Jainism, influencing Asian attitudes and offering a unique perspective on the role of animals in the drama of human life."

This unique perspective is summarized by the well-known exiled leader of the Tibetan people, Tenzin Gyatso, the 14th Dalai Lama, who may well be considered one of the world's most important contemporary religious figures and an eloquent representative of all Eastern nations:

> In our approach to life, be it pragmatic or otherwise, a basic fact that confronts us squarely and unmistakably is the desire for peace, security, and happiness. Different forms of life at different levels of existence make up the teeming denizens of this earth of ours. And, no matter whether they belong to the higher groups such as human beings or to the lower groups such as the animals, all beings primarily seek peace, comfort, and security. Life is as dear to a mute creature as it is to a man. Even the lowliest insect strives for protection against dangers that threaten its life. Just as each one of us wants happiness and fears pain, just as each one of us wants to live and not to die, so do all other creatures [Tenzin Gyatso, *Universal Responsibility and the Good Heart* (Dharmasala, India, Library of Tibetan Works and Archives, 1980), p. 78.]

Western schools of thought are now echoing their parent faiths of the East. As is natural for an adolescent, the young traditions of the West are often extreme in their support of newly found causes. Animal rights and vegetarianism are not exceptions to the rule. Because we are unaccustomed to the sensibility of the *ahimsa* principle and because our own scriptures have been adjusted for reasons already noted, we must grab tightly to our parents' hands and be led gently down the road of truth.

The Golden Rule, "Do unto others as you would have others do unto you," is one of the uniting principles in the world's major religious traditions. In Judaism, it is taught, "What is hateful to you, do not to your fellowmen." (*Talmud, Shabbat,* 31a) Christianity teaches, "Whatever ye would that men should do to you, do ye even so to them." (*Matthew* 7:12) The followers of Islam declare, "No one of you is a believer until he desires for his brother that which he desires for himself." (*Sunnah, Hadith*) In

Confucianism it is said, "Surely it is the maxim of loving kindness: Do not unto others that which you would not have them do unto you." (*Analects* 15.23) Buddhism also teaches, "Hurt not others in ways that you yourself would find hurtful." (*Udana-Varga* 5.18) And finally, in the world's earliest religious scriptures, the Vedic literature, we find, "This is the sum of duty: Do naught unto others which would cause you pain if done to you." (*Mahabharata* 5.1517)

The world of science echoes the world's religions with its own equivalent of The Golden Rule. Newton's Third Law of Motion says that "For every action, there is an equal and opposite reaction." While Newton's Law applies only to material nature, the implications run deeper still, extending to the most subtle levels of existence. In the East, this is called the law of karma.

In a very fundamental sense, too, this law relates to our treatment of animals. The violence in society is at least in part the result of our merciless diet and abuse of the natural world around us. In karmic terms, violence begets violence. In dietary terms, you are what you eat.

"There is a connection between the plight of animals and the many crises that humanity faces each day," describes the International Network for Religion and Animals (INRA). "It is not a misperception to contend that it is a lack of humility, compassion and understanding that underlies humankind's inhumanity, be it toward our own kind through oppression, exploitation, war and deliberate torture and slavery, or towards animals and Nature, as evidenced by well-documented suffering of wild and domestic animals in the world today, and the destruction and pollution of the environment. This situation is the antithesis of the basic teachings of all religions, whose scriptures speak of living in reverence for all life as a significant virtue.

"Religion counsels the powerful to be merciful and kind to those weaker than themselves," INRA continues, "and most of humankind is at least nominally religious. But there is a ghastly paradox: far from showing mercy, humanity uses its dominion over other animal species to pen them in cruel close confinement, to trap, club, harpoon them, to poison, mutilate, and shock them in the name of science, to kill them by the billions, and even slowly to blind them in excruciating pain to test cosmetics. Some of these terrible abuses are due to mistaken understandings of religious principles; others, to a failure to apply those principles."

This short book has been a modest endeavor to show that vegetarianism is not merely a diet, or a way of achieving better health, but rather an important tool for the building of true spiritual life. The success of this book would be in helping people see the urgency of vegetarianism and its benefits, both material and spiritual.

Religion as practiced today has, for the most part, minimized the importance of vegetarianism and compassion for animals. This trend is gradually being reversed. For those of us who take up the banner, our duty is to help newcomers adjust rationally and avoid the overzealousness that accompanies new convictions. Through coherent argument and reason, followers of all faiths can come to see universal compassion and its concomitant vegetarianism as a thread uniting their religions.

> **If you enjoyed this book we feel sure you will also enjoy our other titles listed at the back. Take a look now!**

APPENDICES

RADIO INTERVIEW:
VEGETARIANISM AND THE WORLD
RELIGIONS

*A fter the initial release of **Food for the Spirit**, Steven Rosen was invited to speak on WBAI, a progressive radio station which focuses on cutting-edge and controversial issues, on Shelton Walden's World Watch. The interview aired on June 14, 1987.*

WBAI: Welcome to Worldwatch. This week we'll be talking with Steven Rosen, author of the ground-breaking new book, *Food for the Spirit*. In this work, author Rosen tackles the touchy subjects of diet and religion. Tell our BAI listeners, Steve, why you felt religionists should be aware of diet, especially in relation to vegetarianism and animal rights.

SR: Well, I think that everyone—not only religionists—should be aware of the importance of proper diet. In fact it is a biblical command: "And you shall diligently guard your health and life" (Deut. 4:15). It has been documented that vegetarians live longer and live healthier than do meat-eaters. How can one practice one's religion if one's health is on the wane? So, in this way, the Bible asks us to guard our health. Also, you mentioned "animal rights." Actually, there is another tremendously disregarded biblical command in this regard: *tzar baalay hayyim.* This is Hebrew. It is the mandate to have compassion for animals. And it appears throughout the biblical literature. The problem of animal abuse, however, is quite widespread. In the United States alone, every year, more than 5 billion animals are killed for food and 100 million animals are needlessly tortured in laboratory research.

111

WBAI: I've read similar statistics in vegetarian magazines, such as *Vegetarian Times* and *Animals' Agenda.* How can our listeners know that these facts and figures are not the exaggerations of some predisposed group?

SR: They can know by researching the subject for themselves. This is not simply the concern of some special interest group. It's not like you can only find this information in vegetarian magazines. Rather, these things have been documented in such prestigious journals as *The Journal of the American Medical Association, The American Journal of Clinical Nutrition* and *The Borden Review of Nutrition Research.*

WBAI: Okay. But back to religion. Do you think, practically, that this is a religious issue? I mean aren't the subjects of diet and religion like apples and oranges? True, there are koshering laws in the Jewish faith and, I suppose, similar things in the other religions. But overall I think most people would say that religion is a matter of faith, not dietary preference.

SR: That's true. But what if one's dietary preference affected one's faith? For instance, religion deals with ethics, morals, compassion, and mercy. As Isaac Bashevis Singer has said, "How can we pray to God for mercy if we are not willing to extend mercy to others?" And this is just common sense. It is simply unfair that we do not extend our sense of mercy to the animals. This is, as I have quoted earlier, a biblical precept. Yet we tend to ignore biblical precepts that do not strike our fancy.

Can we be willing to change our hearts but not our diet? The two are inseparable. To claim that these can be separated is sheer hypocrisy! Man does not want to be killed—yet he kills. Man does not want to be the victim of injustice—yet he is unjust. This sort of paradox makes a mockery of religion. The genuine religionist becomes god-like or godly. There is a type of saintliness that comes from being truly religious. As he does not want to be killed, he is careful not to kill others. As he does not want to be the "victim" of a given situation, he does not victimize others. And as he wants God to show him mercy, so also is he merciful to those who are weaker than he. This is fundamental, I think, to real religion. If our diet involves violence— we are setting ourselves up for a nasty future. Violence begets violence. This is the law of karma: "For every action, there is an equal and opposite reaction." For this reason, many Eastern traditions embrace vegetarianism. They believe that he who lives by the sword will die by the sword. In the West we say, " as ye sow, so shall ye reap." In actuality, this is the same as karma. Unfortunately, it is rarely extended to the animals or our diet. But in the East it is.

WBAI: Let's start with the Bible. Can you give us a brief synopsis of vegetarianism in the Old Testament? Just a basic outline.

SR: Yes. In the very first chapter of the first book of the Bible, a non-meat diet is recommended. God says "...I have given you every herb-yielding seed which is upon the face of the earth, and in every tree in which is the fruit of a tree-yielding seed—to you it shall be for food." That's Genesis 1:29. So God does not beat around the burning bush, as it were. Right in the beginning, He emphasizes the vegetarian diet.

And then He explains that this original, non-meat diet is "very good." This is an expression He reserves only for the vegetarian diet. Later diets containing meat are referred to as "concessions" as opposed to "very good."

WBAI: Okay. But what about those concessions? Much later, I believe, God allows Noah and his descendants the option to eat meat.

SR: Still, if studied in context, it is obvious that this is a question of God's permissive will versus His preferred will. In other words, God may have allowed this concession. But He never indicated that this diet was preferable. In fact, He seems to indicate rather clearly that it was not.

I think the crucial thing here is to understand exactly what was taking place in the time of Noah. Actually, man had become so depraved that he would eat a limb immediately torn from a living animal. The situation had become so degraded that God had decided to create a great flood. Incidentally, a great flood, as depicted in the Bible, would have undoubtedly destroyed all vegetation—thus, at that time, there was hardly an alternative to animal foods.

Anyway, God did give a concession at that time for eating meat. This occurs in the 9th chapter of Genesis, where God gives permission to man to eat everything that moves. Soon after, however, God says that man should still not eat the blood of animals (and so the complex koshering laws of the Jews came into play...) and soon after that, God reveals a sort of karma that awaits those who slaughter animals: "By their own hands shall ye be slain." (Genesis 9:5)

WBAI: What happened next? Was meat-eating then at least "allowed" for all time?

SR: Well, not exactly, because there was a second attempt at instituting a vegetarian diet among the Jewish people. When the Israelites left Egypt, God provided "manna," a vegetarian substance, for food. Still, even at that time, the people cried out for meat, and God indeed provided it—along with a plague for all who ate the meat.

They died immediately. The Bible makes careful record of this, and in no uncertain terms calls the burial places of those meat-eaters "the graves of lust." Biblical commentators—predisposed to vegetarianism or not—say the graves were so named because those who were buried there had lusted after flesh foods.

WBAI: Steve, I'm just curious. What about "dominion?" Doesn't the Bible give man dominion over the animals?

SR: Indeed it does. But "dominion" was never taken to mean "abuser" or "exploiter." At least not according traditional biblical usage. Rather, the original Hebrew for the word "dominion" is *yirdu,* and it connotes a sort of stewardship, or guardianship. In other words, we are given the command to "care for" our more humbly endowed brothers and sisters—the animals—not to eat them. For instance, a king is said to have dominion over his subjects. But that doesn't mean that he should eat them, or abuse them. No. He must care for them, help them, and even love them.

I would also like to point out that this biblical verse which gives us dominion over the animals appears in Genesis 1:26. The verse recommending a vegetarian diet, which I have quoted earlier, appears in Genesis 1:29. Three verses later. In other words, God gives us dominion over the animals and, only three verses later, prohibits their use for food. Implicitly, the dominion he gives us cannot include using the animals for food.

WBAI: That seems pretty clear. Why, I wonder, don't more religionists turn to vegetarianism? I mean it seems that there is a very strong case for it in the Bible. Maybe it's just arrogance or...

SR: Ignorance. Yes. There is evidence of both. In the Talmud, this arrogant side is explained quite a bit. It is summed up like this: "When man shall become proud in his heart," the Talmud tells us, "remind him that the little fly has preceded him in creation."

Also, the biblical book Ecclesiastes points out, "For that which befalleth the sons of men, befalleth beasts, even one thing befalleth them: As the one dieth, so dieth the other. They all have one breath. So that man hath no pre-eminence above a beast—for all is vanity." It's plain and simple fact: humans in general, especially in the twentieth century, have a perverse sort of prejudice toward the animals, one that is oftentimes unfounded. We think we're superior to them and that this means we can bully them, torture them, and eat them.

Now let us deal with the question of ignorance. Rather than actually studying their scriptures and ancient traditions from which these scriptures arose, many prefer to learn their religion by turning on the TV and watching Jim Baker and other popular evangelists. If people want to learn whether or not vegetarianism is actually consistent with their religion, they should make a serious study. Unfortunately, many are willing to accept whatever interpretation of their religion that the majority accepts. One must develop the ability to distinguish a given spiritual path from the version of it set forth by those who claim to follow it. People must learn their own religious traditions and the scriptures, too.

WBAI: I agree totally. Steve, we've been focusing primarily on the Jewish tradition. I wonder if you could briefly discuss the Christian perspective.

SR: Basically, over the centuries, there has arisen two distinct schools of Christian thought: the Aristotelian-Thomistic school and the Augustinian-Franciscan school.

WBAI: Can you explain the difference and their relation to vegetarianism?

SR: Yes. The Aristotelian-Thomistic school has, as its fundamental basis, the premise that animals are here for our pleasure—they have no purpose of their own. We can eat them, torture them in laboratories—anything. This is almost Cartesian in scope. Unfortunately, modern Christianity tends to embrace this form of their religion.

The Augustinian-Franciscan school, however, teaches that we are all brothers and sisters under God's fatherhood. Based largely on the world view of St. Francis and being Platonic in nature, this school fits very neatly with the vegetarian perspective.

WBAI: Is there any evidence that Jesus was a vegetarian?

SR: Early Greek manuscripts speak of Jesus as "the Nazarene." I'll tell you why this is significant. Later editions of the Bible refer to "Jesus of Nazareth." And this simply means that he comes from that particular town: Nazareth. But research has revealed that this is a poor translation. A more accurate translation is "Jesus the Nazarene." This is significant because it tells us more than merely the town he comes from, more than that he was just from Nazareth. It means he was from a sect called "the Nazarenes." And it is now known that this particular sect followed Essene principles, including vegetarianism.

WBAI: Do any modern Bibles translate it as "the Nazarene"?

SR: Yes. *The Jerusalem Bible* is one example. There are others. The point is this: he is definitely called "the Nazarene" in many places in the New Testament. So if you wanted to prove that he himself was a vegetarian, this would be a pretty convincing way to prove it. The Nazarenes were definitely vegetarians!

WBAI: Interesting. I was just reading in your book that many early Christian fathers were vegetarian. Historically, has that held true for many prominent Christians?

SR: *The Clementine Homilies*, which was written early in the second century and was based on the teachings of St. Peter, Jesus's direct follower, categorically condemns all kinds of meat-eating and abuse of animals. Clement of Alexandria and even John Wesley, the founder of Methodism, were said to be vegetarians.

There is also a large body of literature devoted to proving that the original Apostles shunned the use of flesh foods, and one can read more about that in my book. The importance of establishing what the early Christians ate is considerable. It's crucial to my case, wouldn't you say?

WBAI: Definitely. It would indicate just what Christians today should eat. At least it would give us an idea...

SR: That's right. In addition, it would give us more of an indication as to Jesus's dietary preferences.

WBAI: Right. Folks, I just want to urge you to go out and buy this book. It's just about the best book on the subject. *Food for the Spirit*, by author Steven Rosen. It also has a preface by Nobel laureate Isaac Bashevis Singer.

Steve, let's get into Eastern religion for a while. Vegetarianism, I know, is deeply ingrained in the Eastern way of thinking, especially in India. Isn't that true?

SR: Oh, definitely! In 1857, when the British introduced their new Enfield rifle to the troops in Bengal, there was a great mutiny. Do you know why this occurred, this great, historic mutiny?

WBAI: No, why?

SR: Because that new Enfield rifle utilized an ammunition cartridge which was coated with animal grease. And the sepoys, as these Bengali troops were called, had to bite off the tip of the cartridge before it was inserted into the rifle. Instead of conforming to this simple procedure, they mutinied. This is how deeply ingrained vegetarianism is in India.

WBAI: Where did this dedication to the meatless way of life begin? I know the origins of Indian religion are shrouded in antiquity. But, still there must be some ancient practice or principle that India's modern day vegetarianism can attributed to...

SR: Well, a lot of it has, as its fundamental basis, cow protection...

WBAI: Oh, yes, how did that come about?

SR: This can be attributed to the worship of Lord Krishna, who is always depicted as a cowherder. Although the Hindu pantheon is multifaceted, originally, Krishna-worship permeated the Vedic, or ancient Indian, tradition. And Krishna is glorified as being particularly fond of *brahmanas*, or those living beings who impart spiritual knowledge to others, and the cows, who give milk to their own calves and to the human race.

The cow is not worshiped in India, as is generally supposed. Rather, she is simply honored as a type of mother—because she gives milk as one's natural mother does. So for this reason, and because she is dear to Krishna—the Supreme Lord—she is, in a sense, revered. Or, at least, greatly respected.

WBAI: What about Mahatma Gandhi? Although he was a great, outspoken vegetarian, I had heard that he was inconsistent in many ways. Can you elaborate on that for a moment?

SR: I don't know if I, as a rule, would accuse Gandhi of inconsistency. After all, he was a deeply religious man and a devout vegetarian as well. Still, I have heard, probably, the same accusations as the ones you are referring to. It has been said that Gandhi was a saint among politicians—but that he was a politician among saints. Anyway, overall, I think, he set a very good example of how one can be religious and a vegetarian at the same time.

WBAI: Since we don't have a lot of time left, maybe you could briefly explain to our BAI listeners why Eastern religions seem to be more conscious of the religious vegetarian imperative. Buddhism, Hinduism, Jainism—they all seem to immediately conjure up a religion of peace and harmlessness. Whereas the Judaeo-Christian tradition seems more shallow, at least in this particular area. Do you have anything to say about this?

SR: As I've written in *Food for the Spirit*, the Eastern traditions promote *sarva-bhuta-hita* ("devotion to the good of all creatures") over *loka-hita* ("devotion for the good of humanity"). The first ethical system, says the Vedic literature, includes the second, and therefore it is more complete. If one cares for all living creatures, one naturally cares for humanity as well—of necessity. The Vedic viewpoint states that one should see the same life-force in all living entities—regardless of outer dress (the body).

Those who cannot understand the principle of life in animals may then eventually misunderstand what the life-force is altogether and lose their sense of humanity. For this reason, *sarva-bhuta-hita* is the superior code of ethics delineated in the Eastern trtaditions. It is, of course, my contention that all the major world religions acknowledged the superior, all-inclusive *sarva-bhuta-hita* at one time or another. Unfortunately, in the West, especially, this truth has been compromised by less intelligent or otherwise ill-informed religious leaders throughout the centuries. It is my prayer that *Food for the Spirit* may give religious people today some food for thought.

WBAI: Well, Steven, I want to sincerely thank you for coming on our show. And I want to say that your presentation is certainly effective in helping people see vegetarianism as a religious imperative. It has helped me in this direction. That's for sure. So, thank you very much.

SR: Thank you.

QUOTES FROM
SCRIPTURES AND SAGES

Judaism and Christianity

"The Lord is good to all, and compassionate toward all His works."
—Psalms 145.9

"The just man takes care of his beast, but the heart of the wicked is merciless."—Proverbs 12.10

"...And the fruit thereof shall be for meat, and the leaf thereof for medicine."—Ezekiel 47.12

"I am full of the burnt offering of rams and the fat of fed beasts, and I delight not in the blood of bullocks, or of lambs, or of the goats..."
—Isaiah 1.11

"When you make many prayers, I will hear not: your hands are full of blood."
—Isaiah 1.15

"I will have mercy, and not sacrifice."—Hosea 6.6

"Be not among the winebibbers; nor among the riotous eaters of flesh!"
—Proverbs 23.20

"He that killeth an ox is as if he slew a man."—Isaiah 66.3

"Thou shalt not kill."—Exodus 20.13

"Thanks be to God: since I gave up flesh and wine, I have been delivered from all physical ills."—John Wesley (1703-1791), founder of Methodism

"Cruelty to animals is as if man did not love God."—Cardinal John H. Newman

"Plant life instead of animal food is the keystone of regeneration. Jesus used bread instead of flesh and wine in place of blood at the Lord's Supper."—Richard Wagner (1813-1883), German composer

Islam

"There is not an animal on the earth, nor a flying creature flying on two wings, but they are peoples like unto you."—Koran, surah 6, verse 38

"Therewith He causes crops to grow for you, and the olive and the date-palm and grapes and all kinds of fruit. Lo! Herein is indeed a portent for people who reflect."—Koran, surah 16, verse 11

"...but to hunt...is forbidden you, so long as ye are on the pilgrimage. Be mindful of your duty to Allah, unto Whom you will all be gathered."
—Koran, surah 5, verse 96

"A token unto them is the dead earth. We revive it, and We bring forth from it grain—so that they will eat thereof. And We have placed therein gardens of the date-palm and grapes, and We have caused springs of water to gush forth therein. That they may eat of the fruit thereof, and their hands created it not. Will they not, then, give thanks?"—Koran, surah 36, verses 33-35

"Maim not the brute beasts."—Prophet Mohammed

"Whoever is kind to the lesser creatures is kind to himself."
—Prophet Mohammed

Buddhism

"To avoid causing terror to living beings, let the disciple refrain from eating meat...the food of the wise is that which is consumed by the sadhus [holymen]; it does not consist of meat...There may be some foolish people in the future who will say that I permitted meat-eating and that I partook of meat myself, but...meat-eating I have not permitted to anyone, I do not permit, I will not permit meat-eating in any form, in any manner and in any place; it is unconditionally prohibited for all."
—Buddha, from the Dhammapada

"He who, seeking his own happiness, punishes or kills beings who also long for happiness, will not find happiness after death."— Dhammapada

"Because he has pity on every living creature, therefore a man is called 'holy.'"—Dhammapada

Hinduism

"The greatness of a nation and its moral progress can be measured by the way in which its animals are treated."—Mahatma Gandhi

"If one has a strong desire for meat, he may make an animal out of clarified butter, or one of flour, and eat that. But let him never seek to destroy a living being..."—Manusmriti 5.37.174

"A cruel and wretched person who maintains his existence at the cost of others' lives deserves to be killed for his own eternal well-being, otherwise he will go down by his own actions."—Shrimad Bhagavatam 1.7.37

"Everything is related. Whatever happens now to animals will eventually happen to man."—Indira Gandhi

"As long as human society continues to allow cows to be regularly killed in slaughterhouses, there cannot be any question of peace and prosperity."
—A. C. Bhaktivedanta Swami Prabhupada

Miscellaneous

"It is my view that the vegetarian manner of living, by its purely physical effect on the human temperament, would most beneficially influence the lot of mankind."—Albert Einstein

"O my fellow men, do not defile your bodies with sinful foods....The earth affords a lavish supply of riches, of innocent foods, and offers you banquets that involve no bloodshed or slaughter."—Pythagoras, from *Metamorphoses* by Ovid

"As long as men massacre animals, they will kill each other. Indeed, he who sows the seeds of murder and pain cannot reap joy and love."
—Pythagoras

"Truly man is the king of beasts, for his brutality exceeds them. We live by the death of others. We are burial places! I have since an early age abjured the use of meat..."—Leonardo Da Vinci

"When a man wants to murder a tiger, he calls it sport; when a tiger wants to murder him, he calls it ferocity."—George Bernard Shaw

"Educate the children in their infancy in such a way that they become exceedingly kind and merciful to the animals."—'Abdul-Baha; Baha'i World Faith

"I do not see any reason why animals should be slaughtered to serve as human diet when there are so many substitutes. After all, man can live without meat..."—The Dalai Lama

"A dead cow or sheep lying in a pasture is recognized as carrion. The same sort of a carcass dressed and hung up in a butcher's stall passes as food!"
—J. H. Kellogg

"Every act of irreverence for life, every act which neglects life, which is indifferent to and wastes life, is a step towards the love of death. This choice man must make at every minute. Never were the consequences of the wrong choice as total and as irreversible as they are today. Never was the warning of the Bible so urgent: 'I have put before you life and death, blessing and curse. Choose life, that you and your children may live.' (Deuteronomy 30:19)"—Erich Fromm

SELECT BIBLIOGRAPHY

Adams, Carol J., *The Sexual Politics of Meat: A Feminist-Vegetarian Critical Theory* (New York: Continuum, 1990).

Alladin, Bilkiz, *The Story of Mohammed the Prophet* (India, Hemkunt Press, 1979).

Altman, Nathaniel, *Eating for Life* (Wheaton, Il., Quest Books, 1973).

————*Ahimsa: Dynamic Compassion* (Wheaton, Il., Quest Books, 1980).

Ausubel, Nat, *The Book of Jewish Knowledge* (New York, Crown Pub., 1964).

Barnard, Neal, *Eat Right, Live Longer* (New York: Harmony Books, 1995).

————*Food for Life* (New York: Crown, 1993).

Berman, Louis, *Vegetarianism and Jewish Tradition* (New York, KTAV Pub., 1981).

Berry, Rynn, *The New Vegetarians* (New York: Pythagorean Publishers, 1993).

————*Famous Vegetarians & Their Recipes* (Los Angeles: Panjandrum Books, 1990).

Chapple, Christopher, K., *Nonviolence to Animals, Earth, and Self in Asian Traditions* (Albany: State University of New York Press, 1993).

Cook, John, *Diet and Your Religion* (New York, Woodbridge Press, 1976).

Dasa, Adiraja, *The Hare Krishna Book of Vegetarian Cooking* (Paris, The Bhaktivedanta Book Trust, 1984).

Dombrowski, Daniel A., *The Philosophy of Vegetarianism* (Amherst, University of Mass. Press, 1984).

Dresner, Rabbi Samuel H., *The Jewish Dietary Laws: Their Meaning for our Time* (New York, Burning Bush Press, 1959).

Ferrier, Rev. J. Todd, *On Behalf of the Creatures* (England, The Order of the Cross, 1968).

Freedman, Rabbi Seymour E., *The Book of Kashruth* (New York, Bloch Publishing Co., 1970).

Giehl, Dudley, *Vegetarianism: A Way of Life*, foreword by Isaac Bashevis Singer, (New York, Harper & Row, 1979).

Golden, Hyman E., *A Jew and His Duties* (New York, Hebrew Publishing Co., 1953).

Head, Joseph, and Cranston, S. L., *Reincarnation: The Phoenix Fire Mystery* (New York, Warner Books, 1977).

Holmes-Gore, Rev. V. A., *These We Have Not Loved* (England, The C. W. Daniel Company Ltd., 1946).

Hume, C. H., *The Status of Animals in the Christian Religion* (England, University Federation for Animal Welfare, 1957).

Kalechofsky, Roberta, ed., *Judaism and Animal Rights: Classical and Contemporary Responses* (Marblehead, Massachusetts: Micah Publications, 1993).

————*Haggadah for the Liberated Lamb* (Marblehead, Mass., Micah Pub., 1985).

Kapleau, Philip, *To Cherish All Life: The Buddhist Case for Becoming Vegetarian* (New York, Harper & Row, 1981).

Khaki, MI, "An Article on Islam and Vegetarianism" (Madras, The Vegetarian Way, 1977).

Khan, Ghulam Mustafa, *Al-Dhabh: Slaying Animals for Food the Islamic Way* (London, Ta Ha Pub., 1982).

Lappe, Frances Moore, *Diet for a Small Planet* (New York, Ballantine Books, 1975).

Lebeau, Rabbi James M., *The Jewish Dietary Laws: Sanctify Life* (New York, United Synagogue of America, 1983).

Linzey, Andrew, *Animal Theology* (Illinois: University of Illinois Press, 1995).

———*Christianity and the Rights of Animals* (New York: Crossroad, 1987).

———*Animal Rights: A Christian Assessment of Man's Treatment of Animals* (London, SCM Press, Ltd., 1976).

———*The Status of Animals in the Christian Tradition* (England, Woodbrooke College, 1985).

Mahmud, Abdel H., *The Creed of Islam* (England, World of Islam Festival Trust, 1978).

Moran, Victoria, *Compassion: The Ultimate Ethic* (England, Thorsons Pub., 1985).

Muhaiyaddeen, Muhammad Rahim Bawa, *Come to the Secret Garden* (Philadelphia, PA, The Fellowship Press, 1985).

———*Asma'ul-Husna: The 99 Beautiful Names of Allah* (Philadelphia, PA, The Fellowship Press, 1979).

Parham, Barbara, *What's Wrong With Eating Meat?*(Colorado, Ananda Marg Pub., 1979).

Porphyry, *On Abstinence from Animal Food,* trans. from the Greek by Thomas Taylor, ed. Esme Wynne-Tyson, (London, Cantaur, Boston, Brandon, 1965).

Prabhupada, A. C. Bhaktivedanta Swami, *Bhagavad-gita As It Is* (Los Angeles, Collier-Macmillan, 1972).

———*Chaitanya Charitamrita,* 17 vols., (Los Angeles, Bhaktivedanta Book Trust, 1975).

———*The Path of Perfection* (Los Angeles, Bhaktivedanta Book Trust, 1979).

———*Shrimad Bhagavatam,* Cantos 1-10, 30 vols., (New York/Los Angeles, Bhaktivedanta Book Trust, 1972-80).

Quarelli, Elena, *Socrates and the Animals,* trans. by Kathleen Speight (London, Hodder and Stoughton, 1960).

Regan, Tom, *The Case for Animal Rights* (California, University of California Press, 1983).

———*Animal Sacrifices: Religious Perspectives on the Use of Animals in Science* (Philadelphia, PA, Temple University Press, 1986).

Regan, Tom, and Singer, Peter, ed., *Animal Rights and Human Obligations* (New Jersey, Prentice-Hall Inc., 1976).

Regenstein, Lewis, G., *Replenish the Earth* (New York: The Crossroad Publishing Company, 1991).

Reyes, Benito F., *Scientific Evidence for the Existence of the Soul* (Wheaton, Il., Quest Books, 1970).

Rifkin, Jeremy, *Beyond Beef: The Rise and Fall of the Cattle Culture* (New York: Dutton, 1992).

Rice, Pamela, *101 Reasons Why I'm a Vegetarian* (New York: The Viva Vegie Society, 1996).

Robbins, John, *Diet for a New America* (Wapole, N.H.: Stillpoint Publishing, 1987).

Rollin, Bernard E., *Animal Rights and Human Morality* (New York, Prometheus Books, 1981).

Rudd, Geoffrey L., *Why Kill for Food?* (Madras, India, The Indian Vegetarian Congress, 1956).

Ruesch, Hans, *Slaughter of the Innocent* (New York, Bantam Books, 1978).

Saddhatissa, H., *The Life of the Buddha* (New York, Harper & Row, 1976).

Sanehi, Swaran Singh, "Vegetarianism in Sikhism" (Madras, The Vegetarian Way, 1977).

Schochet, Elijah Judah, *Animal Life in Jewish Tradition* (New York, KTAV Pub., 1984).

Schwartz, Richard, *Judaism and Vegetarianism* (New York, Exposition Press, 1982).

Siddiqi, Muhammad Iqbal, *The Ritual of Animal Sacrifice in Islam* (Pakistan, Kasi Pub., 1982).

Singer, Peter, *Animal Liberation* (New York, Avon Pub., 1975).

Smith, Scott, "Vegetarianism and Christianity" in *Vegetarian Times* (April 1981).

Sussman, Vic, *The Vegetarian Alternative* (PA, Rodale Press, 1978).

Suzuki, Dr. Daisetz T., *The Chain of Compassion* (Cambridge, MA, Cambridge Buddhist Association, 1966).

Syed, Dr. M. Hafiz, *Thus Spoke Muhammed* (Madras, Amra Press, 1962).

Tahtinen, Unto, *Ahimsa: Non-violence in the Indian Tradition* (London, Rider & Co., 1976).

Tannahill, Reay, *Food in History* (New York, Stein and Day Pub., 1973).

Vedic Contemporary Library Series, *The Higher Taste* (Los Angeles, CA, Bhaktivedanta Book Trust, 1983).

Wynne-Tyson, Jon, *Food For A Future: The Complete Case for Vegetarianism* (London, Centaur Press, 1979).

INDEX

ABOUT THE AUTHOR

For the past 25 years, Steven Rosen has been both a devout vegetarian and an eloquent advocate of the vegetarian ideal. His articles and books have appeared in several languages and he is a frequent contributor to such publications as *Vegetarian Times, The Minaret* (a quarterly Islamic newspaper), *Back to Godhead* (a bi-monthly magazine of Vedic culture and spirituality), and *Wie Es Ist* (a German philosophical journal.) After completing his studies in Hebrew and Biblical literature in New York City, he undertook several extensive tours of the Indian subcontinent, exploring vegetarianism as espoused in Eastern religion and culture.

Steven J. Rosen is a freelance writer and author of 11 books, including *East-West Dialogues* and *Om Shalom.* Currently, he is editor of the *Journal of Vaishnava Studies,* an academic quarterly that is highly regarded and supported by scholars throughout the world.

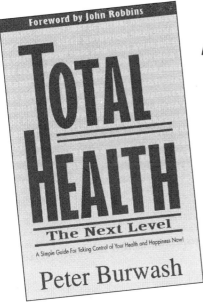

by Peter Burwash
Foreword by John Robbins

$11.95 ISBN #1-887089-10-1
6"x 9", paper 156 pgs.

"Read **Total Health** and heed its
wise and compassionate counsel,
and you will be well on the way to
new levels of aliveness, healing
and joy."

John Robbins, Author,
Diet for a New America

Total Health: The Next Level

A Simple Guide For Taking Control of Your Health and Happiness Now!

Exploding the Myths of America's Diet and Exercise Programs

Most of us put health and vitality at the top of our goal lists. But we have a hard time achieving it. Despite having so much information at our fingertips and the presence of enormous nutrition, diet and exercise industries enticing us with promises, most of us find remaining committed to a healthy life style a losing battle. Why?

For more than 20 years Peter Burwash has been answering this question and teaching people around the world the simple truths of how to finally reach their goals of health and happiness. He explains with simplicity and compassion how our food and life style choices have a life-changing impact not only on our own future, health and happiness, but that of the entire planet.

Total Health is a wonderful gift for friends, loved ones or yourself.
Order your copies today!

Available from your local bookseller, or just fill out the order form in back
and fax it, or call us toll free at:
1-888-TORCHLT (867-2458) Fax: (209) 337-2354

The Vegetarian Revolution

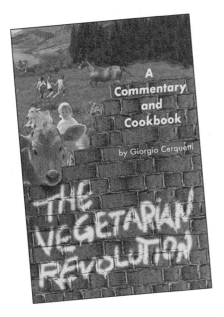

by Giorgio Cerquetti

$11.95 ISBN #1-887089-00-4
6"x 9", paper 184 pgs.

"...it is not only fascinating, fun and engrossing, it has the potential—if its message is heeded—to literally save the world. This is a must read for everyone concerned about the fate of our planet and what we can do to save it."

Lewis Regenstein, Author,
Replenishing The Earth

Join The Peaceful Revolution!

Famous vegetarians, from ancient through modern times, lend their powerful voices to an idea whose time has come. *The Vegetarian Revolution* is a revealing presentation of precise, detailed and convincing reasons why humankind should move toward adopting a vegetarian diet. You'll enjoy the 108 delicious favorite recipes and compelling quotes gathered from renowned vegetarian gourmet chefs, celebrities, artists, spiritual leaders and noted vegetarians of the past.

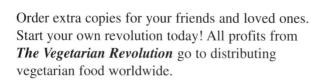

Order extra copies for your friends and loved ones. Start your own revolution today! All profits from *The Vegetarian Revolution* go to distributing vegetarian food worldwide.

Available from your local bookseller, or just fill out the order form in back and fax it, or call us toll free at:
1-888-TORCHLT (867-2458) Fax: (209) 337-2354

The Reincarnation Controversy

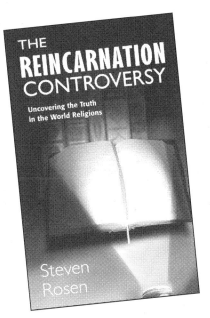

by Steven Rosen

$11.95 ISBN #1-887089-11-X
6"x 9", paper 140 pgs.

"...Rosen clears up many myths and stereotypes of reincarnationist thought found in the major world religions. It is a pleasure to see so many sources collected and summarized into a nice, small volume, which will be effective in educating students and public readers alike."

Guy L. Beck, Ph.D.,
Dept. of Religious Studies,
Loyola University

Uncovering the Truth in the World Religions

Is Reincarnation the Gospel Truth?

When people begin to explore the concept of reincarnation as a possible explanation to life's fundamental mysteries, they often turn to their own religious traditions for guidance. In many cases, they encounter explicit rejection of the concept. If they had a chance, however, to explore the history of their own religions, they might be surprised to see that there is no barrier at all to the acceptance of reincarnation.

In *The Reincarnation Controversy*, Steven Rosen gives readers just this chance. He guides us through the history of the world's religions, showing how the teachings of all of them are consistent with the idea of reincarnation. Rosen's scholarly yet readable style makes this book an excellent resource for the general public as well as students of religion.

Order a copy today and begin your journey!

Available from your local bookseller, or just fill out the order form in back and fax it, or call us toll free at:
1-888-TORCHLT (867-2458) Fax: (209) 337-2354

Book Order Form ———————

☎ Telephone orders: Call 1-888-TORCHLT (1-888-867-2458).
Have your VISA or MasterCard ready.

❊ FAX orders: 209-337-2354

✉ Postal orders: Torchlight Publishing   PO Box 52
Badger CA 93603-0052 USA

▲ World Wide Web: www.torchlightpub.com

Please send the following: QTY

• **Total Health**, by Peter Burwash $11.95 x ___ = $ _____

• **The Key to Great Leadership**, by Peter Burwash $9.95 x ___ = $ _____

• **The Vegetarian Revolution**, by Giorgio Cerquetti $11.95 x ___ = $ _____

• **Diet for Transcendence**, by Steven Rosen $11.95 x ___ = $ _____

Sales Tax: (CA residents add 7.75%) . . . .$ _____

S/H (see below) . . . .$ _____

TOTAL . . . . $ _____

◯ Please send me more information on other books published by Torchlight Publishing.

Company: _____

Name: _____

Address: _____

City:_____ State_____ Zip_____

(I understand that I may return any books for a full refund — for any reason, no questions asked.)

Payment:

◯ Check/money order enclosed   ◯ VISA   ◯ MasterCard

Card Number: _____

Name on Card: _____ Exp. date_____

Signature: _____

Shipping and handling:

USA : $3.00 for first book and $1.75 for each additional book. Air mail per book (USA only) — $4.00
Canada : $5.00 for first book and $2.50 for each additional book
Foreign countries: $8.00 for first book, $4.00 for each additional book.
Surface shipping may take 3-4 weeks. Foreign orders please allow 6-8 weeks for delivery.